To the Bolton Medical Society

with best wishes

Idris Williams

Dec 1979.

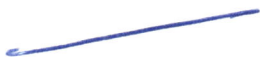

THE CARE OF THE ELDERLY IN THE COMMUNITY

The Care of the Elderly in the Community

IDRIS WILLIAMS

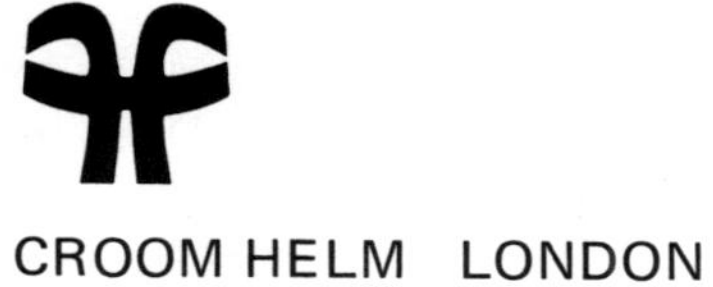

CROOM HELM LONDON

Croom Helm Ltd, 2-10 St John's Road, London SW11

British Library Cataloguing in Publication Data

Williams, Idris
The care of the elderly in the community.
1. Aged – Great Britain – Care and hygiene
I. Title
362.6'0941 HV1481.G5

ISBN 0-85664-789-6
ISBN 0-85664-708-X Pbk

Printed in Great Britain by offset lithography by
Billing & Sons Ltd, Guildford, London and Worcester

CONTENTS

TABLES

FIGURES

To my elderly patients and friends,
many of whom are shining examples of
successful living in old age.

PREFACE

My interest in old people began in 1968. By that time I had already been in general practice for over ten years. Wherever I had worked, I inherited or quickly acquired what was called a chronic visiting list, which consisted in the main of persons over 65 years. Some were housebound and had a chronic illness which needed supervision; but others I visited came to expect and even demand their monthly call. Over the years I slowly became aware of a number of things: first, that many of the patients I visited routinely were quite mobile and went out for almost all of their other requirements (indeed often went straight to the chemist's shop after my visit); secondly, that I was coming across patients with acute problems, whom I had not previously seen and who ought to have been visited earlier; thirdly, I was impressed by the high incidence of anaemia in the old people. I therefore decided with the help of my partners to see every patient over 75 years and test their blood for anaemia. When planning this exercise we became aware of the work of James Williamson and his colleagues in Edinburgh on unreported need amongst the elderly. Their now classic article had been published four years previously. The work they did had been carried out on patients of 65 years and over who were partly selected from three general practices. We therefore decided to extend our own survey to a full medical and social assessment of our very old patients and to attempt to see each one in the practice and assess unreported need. The first surprise was the number of very old people we were responsible for. From a list of 7,200 patients we had 340 who were over 75 years old. I had been battling manfully to see about 40 of these a month (or at least 40 of the much larger number of over-65s). A major research exercise developed and was supported by a DHSS grant. The subsequent story has been told in many published papers, and much of the technical information gathered was written up by me as part of an MD thesis in 1973.

The study changed my attitude to the care of old people. The tedious chore of a chronic visiting list disappeared and a much more positive and interesting idea replaced it. By screening, I discover those old people who are at risk and need surveillance by either myself or the health visitor. Those who can come to the surgery are encouraged to do so and although I still visit many old people regularly, I am much happier that my visits are really necessary. I also know much more about the lives of my old patients and what they themselves want and expect from the medical and social services. A high percentage are happy, fully integrated members of society who live interesting lives. Indeed, I have enjoyed listening to and learning from the many remarkable characters who have turned up at our screening clinics. Their philosophy, considering some of the events which have happened to them during their long lives, has often been deeply moving. I was impressed by the successful living many were achieving even in advanced old age.

I therefore became interested in the quality of life after the age of 75 and felt convinced that I should be contributing to it. I rejected the nihilistic attitude adopted by many which asserts that nothing can be done to help old age and that to intervene is worthless. As one doctor put it: 'Why bother to wake a hungry man to tell him that there is no food available?' I maintain, however, that much can be done. A great deal has been learned about the ageing process and the difficulties experienced by the elderly; and it is now realised that help is possible to overcome many of these problems. These can be medical or social and sometimes a combination of both. It has been clear for some time that helping people through these situations involves a team of workers. The primary health care team comes into its own when looking after the elderly, but really needs extending to include social workers. The aim should really be to have a community care team to provide a comprehensive service.

Having said this, it is however necessary to introduce a caveat. The provision of services must not in a sense be the principal objective when considering care for the elderly. The main aim must be to keep old people self-supportive and independent. It would be wrong if as a result of intervention self-reliance were lost. Obviously, help will sometimes be necessary and may be on a long-term basis, but wherever possible a return to self-sufficiency should be the aim. The wishes of the aged themselves must always be respected and they must be consulted about their needs. Undoubtedly the independence I have just described is high on their list of priorities.

The aim of this book is therefore to describe domiciliary care in its widest sense for old people. I am not advocating a special geriatric community service, or producing a textbook of geriatrics. The care I visualise is given by the team who also look after the rest of society. Indeed, it is a basic principle that old people should be regarded as part of the community and not segregated and treated as different. They should do the shopping, collect the pension, attend the surgery and so on. But for the over-75s particularly, there are opportunities for prevention, maintenance and rehabilitation which can realistically improve the quality of their lives. This is the aim of care, and will be the major theme of this book.

Another feature which was very apparent in our original studies was the part played by the family in providing care for the elderly. This might be the husband and wife for each other, or often daughters and, occasionally, sisters and brothers. The importance of this care for the type of life lived by old people cannot be over-stressed and there is unfortunately some evidence that this availability may be diminishing. Nevertheless, the family will continue to provide most of the care needed in the community. I had originally thought of writing this book for members of the community care team, but considering the importance of the family I have tried to make it readable and informative to someone who might be looking after an elderly relative. There are therefore three different types of reader – the professional carers (doctors, nurses, social workers, physiotherapists, occupational therapists, speech therapists and, indeed, all members of the team); the students of these professions; and family members and other interested lay people such as voluntary workers and reception staff at surgeries or health centres. I realise in aiming at so wide a group of readers, I may not satisfy any one of them. The danger is obvious but as so many people are involved in looking after the aged, I thought the risk worth taking. As medical terms sometimes cause difficulty, a glossary has been included.

I have adopted throughout a practical approach to the subject and the topics chosen will, I hope, be helpful to those engaged in looking after old people outside hospital and are based very much on my own experience. I have occasionally over-simplified, but where this has happened, I have suggested some further reading at the end of the chapter. I have also inevitably had to be selective. Some chapters are more technical than others but even so, it is hoped that they will be of interest to lay readers. The chapters on the social status of old people and the social problems they experience are not meant to be a full account of the subject, but rather an introduction that can be followed up in more detailed textbooks.

I am indebted to many people for help and encouragement during the preparation of this book and I would particularly like to record my gratitude to Dr Martin Garland, Dr David Jolley, Dr Peter O'Loughlin, Dr Brice Pitt, Dr Alistair Roddie, Dr Peter Anderson, Dr Arip Benerjee,

Dr David Orrell, Dr Graham Griffiths, Professor J.C. Brocklehurst and Professor P.R.J. Burch, Janet Davidson, Eileen Fairhurst, Dorothy Murfin, John Roe, Chris Perry, David Matthews, J.B. Bamforth, Peter Hope and A.C. Bebbington, for their help with criticising chapters and checking technical information. My partners, Frances Bennett and Peter Saul, have put up with a great deal when I have been writing and have taken more than their fair share of the practice work. To them I am deeply grateful.

I would like to express a special word of thanks to Jim Leeming who, during the past ten years, has kindled in me an interest in old people, and who has always been generous with his help, time and advice. His criticisms and encouragement have been very welcome. He undertook the task of reading the whole script and his many suggestions have improved the end product significantly.

I would also like to thank my secretary, Mrs Lila Fairclough, for her continuing support and loyalty. Her typing skill is legendary and without her help I doubt whether the book would ever have been produced.

Finally, I would like to thank my wife and daughters for living with 'the book' for so long. Their help has been deeply appreciated. Diana and Sarah have read through and suggested changes in the text and Mary has prepared the charts and figures.

Idris Williams

PART ONE: GENERAL BACKGROUND TO AGEING

This section sets the scene of present-day life in old age. It starts however, with an historical account of the evolution of care for old people, so that the pattern of contemporary services and the standard of life experienced can be seen in perspective. A brief look is taken at certain demographical trends which are critically important when planning for the needs of old people both now and in the future.

The following two chapters look at the physical and social status of the elderly. The natural history of ageing is described, including the changes which occur both physically and mentally and the different characteristics and presentations of illness. Over the past decade new insights have been obtained into the significance of certain behavioural traits in elderly people. An example is the phenomenon of non-reporting of illness. The importance of functional ability rather than the presence or absence of disease is also now well recognised. These are described in this section which is, in essence, an account of the factors which set the tone to the quality of life experienced by old people.

1 HISTORICAL

Little is known about the way in which primitive societies cared for their old people and how many members of these ancient communities survived into old age to achieve perhaps the venerated and respected position of village elder. In more recent times, old people have always been a feature of society and, indeed, the services currently available for their care, both in hospital and in the community, are directly linked to events in the past. The story of the development of these services is complicated by the fact that at least four different features of old age have needed help and understanding. These have been, the process of ageing, disease, poverty, and social neglect. The solutions of the resultant problems have been achieved in different ways and they have rarely occurred simultaneously. The history of the attempts made to tackle the last three features is really that of the development of medical and social care for the whole of society. When improvements take place in the standard of care in the community itself, the elderly also benefit; but the old also have had special hazards linked with the ageing process and this has shown itself especially in the degree to which they are unable to care for themselves. A new development is the increase in numbers of old people and the impact caused by this has yet to be faced.

Ageing and Disease

It seems that the differentiation of the two separate processes of ageing and disease has long caused confusion. Hippocrates, writing in the fourth century BC, believed that the process of ageing was due to a progressive loss of the body reserves of innate heat and the resultant loss of vitality accounted not only for the fact that old people often had pneumonia without any rise in temperature, but also for their generally increased susceptibility to illness.[1]

These ideas led to the conclusion that ageing itself was a disease. Galen (AD 131-200) challenged this view and did not accept that ageing and disease were synonymous. His insight was remarkable, and to illustrate this, Brian Livesley,[2] writing on the historical aspects of ageing and disease, quotes the following passage from a translation of Galen's *Hygiene*:

> Nor is weakness of function strictly speaking a disease. . .one ought not, therefore, to determine health and disease merely by vigour or weakness of function; but one should apply to the healthy the term 'in accordance with nature' and to the sick the term 'contrary to nature', and disease a condition producing function contrary to nature.[3]

Nevertheless, the Hippocratic view seems to have prevailed despite the fascination which the subject obviously had for philosophers and scientists. They were interested primarily, of course, in achieving longevity, and much advice was given as to how this could be attained. Livesley quotes Roger Bacon, the Franciscan Friar (1214-92), advising 'mirth, singing and looking on human beauty and comeliness' as a method of restraining, retarding and driving away old age.[4] Although he failed to distinguish between old age and disease, Bacon at least appeared to understand much about human nature.

With the gradual increase in the population from the fifteenth century onwards and the introduction of Renaissance thinking, the influence of Galen grew. His advice on general hygiene and moderation was accepted by physicians and they began to appreciate that ageing and disease in old age were separate processes. But it was not until late in the nineteenth century that the principles of diagnosis and treatment of these diseases were finally being established. It was early in the present century that the term 'geriatrics' (*geron* – old man, *iatrikos* – medical treatment) was invented by the American physician Ignaz Nascher, and even then it was some time before specialised medical care for old people came to be universally established and adopted.[5] The problem of the chronically ill elderly was not taken seriously, and, as has been stated by J.H. Sheldon, 'these people were herded into workhouse infirmaries without any attempt made at classification of illness, and virtually none at treatment.'[6] It was into this type of situation of medical neglect and social squalor that Marjorie Warren arrived when she went to work at the West Middlesex Hospital in Isleworth in 1935. Her dedication to the care and treatment of old people in her charge led to the establishment of geriatric medicine as a discipline. Many pioneer geriatricians followed her example and tackled the problems of the elderly sick in hospital. Geriatric departments were founded in most general hospitals. Academic acceptance of geriatric medicine was achieved by the setting up of university chairs in the subject. The first was at Glasgow where W. Ferguson Anderson was appointed Professor of Geriatric Medicine and this example was followed by many other universities.

As well as the clinical discipline of geriatrics, the study of ageing itself has also achieved recognition with the formation of the science of gerontology. In this country early contributions were made by such people as Vladimir Korenchevsky at the Oxford Gerontological Institute, Sir Peter Medawar and Dr Alex Comfort, and research is now proceeding at many centres. The twin problems of disease and the effect of ageing have thus been tackled by doctors and scientists and although much yet remains to be achieved, considerable progress has been made into their management and understanding.

The Relief of Social Neglect and Poverty

Social neglect and poverty have been tackled in a different way. Until the Middle Ages, the churches had been the main source of help for both the poor and the elderly. In the eight century, for example, the Archbishop of York instructed his clergy to collect tithes and set aside one-third of the total for the use of the poor, a category which included many elderly people.[7] In the Middle Ages there was theoretically no welfare problem and the feudal system made the landed aristocracy responsible for the welfare of their inferiors.[8] The Crown itself looked after its servants and several hospitals were founded in this way. The Church also founded hospitals and almshouses, many of which are still in existence at the present time. Later, the parish assumed some broader functions, and rates were levied to relieve the needs of the poor. Little discrimination was made initially between the different types of people who needed help. Monasteries gave food to anyone who asked and as well as the elderly, vagrants and beggars also benefited. As time progressed, government began to move slowly towards the realisation that poverty might not be due only to idleness, but also to old age, disability, and an increasing number of people being deprived of their traditional employment by changing economic circumstances.

By the sixteenth century the number of agricultural labourers who had to rely on wages alone with no land of their own to supplement their income was increasing. The Tudor government passed a series of Poor Laws, culminating in the famous Poor Law Act of 1601. It was motivated by the need to cope with the problems created by roving bands of poor people, some of them genuinely unemployed, and others composed of ex-servicemen and retainers, who were a potential source of discontent. Poverty was a problem exacerbated by the increase in population, the enclosure of land for sheep rather than arable farming, and a number of bad harvests towards the end of the century. The 1601

Act consolidated the principles of family responsibility for old people and provided a Parish Officer to administer relief to appropriate recipients. At first this was given at home but slowly institutes for indoor care were created. These were primarily for the care of the aged sick and infirm and no able-bodied pauper was admitted. Outdoor relief was still given and was in fact extended by expedients such as the Speenhamland System of 1795 (allowances to vary with the price of bread and the size of the labourer's family) which then became part of the fabric of rural pauperisation. At attempt was made to abolish the outdoor system of relief by the Poor Law Amendment Act of 1834. Poor relief was intended to be found in the newly created workhouse or not at all. However, although the Act was ruthlessly applied in the south of England, it was strongly resisted in the north where it was particularly inappropriate to the fluctuating conditions of industrial employment. By the second half of the nineteenth century, the new Poor Law was almost as subject to local variation as the old Poor Law had come to be in the eighteenth century.

One of the long-term results of the Act was that many workhouses were set up, but in them there was no provision for nursing the sick. The elderly could get medical attention in associated infirmaries if this was needed, but for the able-bodied poor old person there was only the workhouse. The rigours of these establishments created a horror in the minds of old people and made them determined to live independently outside. This was the pattern of care throughout most of the nineteenth century. If old people could not be looked after by their families, or were unable to care for themselves, they went into the workhouse if they were fit and into the infirmary if they were ill. When Joseph and Hannah Brown were too aged and infirm to look after each other, this did not seem to be the solution they wanted or needed, for as Laurie Lee points out in *Cider with Rosie*,

> The workhouse could not give them the mercy they needed, but could only divide them in charity. Much better to hide or die in a ditch or starve in one's familiar kitchen watched by the objects one's life had gathered – the scrubbed, empty table; the plates and saucepans; the cold grates; the white, stopped clock.'[9]

Much has been written about the appalling standards of care in these institutions, and, as has been indicated earlier, these persisted well into the present century. Large numbers of workhouses were built and many are still used to house geriatric departments of district general hospitals.

Unfortunately, old attitudes die hard, and there is still present amongst the elderly a sense of horror at the thought of being admitted to a hospital department which they still associate with the old workhouse. The distinction between ill and healthy old people is now theoretically clear: the hospitals as part of the National Health Service are available for the sick, whereas the able-bodied old person without a home or in social difficulties is the responsibility of the Local Authority and care is provided by Social Service departments in their welfare homes, a responsibility laid down in Section 3 of the 1948 National Assistance Act. The concepts of the role which these two systems should play are changing, and in practice there is considerable overlap between them. Even so, since the 1960s an attempt has been made to define the spheres of activity of health and welfare services.

The problem of providing an adequate income for old people, like that of providing suitable accommodation for them, has also exercised the minds of reformers and legislators in both the nineteenth and twentieth centuries. For instance, in 1890, it was disclosed that a third of all fit persons in the UK over the age of seventy were in receipt of Poor Relief. The idea gained ground that all old people should be entitled to a weekly pension and in 1908 the first Old Age Pensions were introduced. The reaction of old people to this was often one of supreme gratitude, and apparently it was not uncommon for them to take bunches of flowers and cakes to the girls in the Post Office who gave out the money. The story from then until the present day is of gradually increasing provision of Old Age Pensions, although the aim of having this at a high enough level to enable all old people to be free from financial problems is, as yet, not really being achieved. A sizeable proportion of the elderly population is in receipt of Supplementary Benefit, to make up for deficiencies in the present level of Old Age Pension.

Care in the Home

Historically, care in the home has been very firmly in the hands of the family, and medical attention has usually been provided by general practitioners or by the apothecary of earlier times. This pattern of medical care was perpetuated by the National Health Service Act of 1946. Health visiting, domiciliary nursing and general practitioner services were made freely available to all, including the elderly within their own homes. By the 1950s, when geriatric departments were being established, it was also becoming clear that the nursing of many chronically sick old persons was taking place within the community itself. J.H. Sheldon, when calling for more care for old people in hospital, also drew attention to the plight of old people in their own homes.[10] He thought it would be necessary to provide a special medical service for old people, with the aim of preserving independence for as long as possible, and later stated that 7 per cent of old people were imposing on the younger generation strains of such severity that life was robbed of normal meaning.[11] He was impressed by this figure which was not only large but was at least twice and perhaps three times the number already being cared for in institutions (and here he probably meant hospitals) and special homes. Sheldon did not mention the GP as a provider of community care for old people and it was not until much later that the concept of the Primary Health Care Team was advocated.

In recent years, there has been renewed interest in the care of the elderly in the community and new insights into their problems have been gained. Williamson *et al.*, for instance, showed the importance of unreported need, and many GPs have conducted surveys of their patients and have advocated screening clinics to recognise illness in its early stages.[12] Thus, domiciliary care of old people is developing but not yet perhaps on the scale that hospital care did two or three decades ago. There are also contemporary problems which are as yet unsolved. These will be discussed in Chapter 5 and some of the developing patterns of care described in Chapter 7.

Development of Care in Other Countries

It is not only in the UK that there have been problems in caring for old people, for most advanced societies have had to deal with similar situations. The way in which these problems have been solved has varied. Sometimes there has been a gradual evolution of care, as in the USA, but occasionally revolutionary events have taken a hand as in Russia, and to a certain extent in the UK, where the introduction of the National Health Service dramatically altered the resources diverted to medical care and the provisions available. In the Netherlands there has been no development of the medical speciality of geriatrics, although old people are often cared for by specialists in chronic illness. Nursing homes provide specific care for the aged sick and these seem to be a half-way house between the hospital and welfare home. In the USA, the health care system was historically characterised by inequalities which especially affected the old. Medicare legislation has, however, provided unimpeded access to hospital and doctor services for the bulk of the elderly population although financial difficulties remain and indeed the reimbursement arrangements in the US now actually militate against much provision of home care services especially with the lack of home visiting tradition among US doctors. Nursing homes, again, seem to be the main provider of institutional care for the aged and these are basically privately owned. There is often a reciprocal discharge agreement between these homes and nearby hospitals, so that theoretically there is a free exchange of patients dependent on medical and social considerations. Hospital-based community care is also available from some centres, for instance at the Montefiore Hospital in New York City. The provision of home care services seems, however, to be patchy and there are obvious strains when prolonged domiciliary care is necessary for disabled old persons.

In the USSR, the importance of health care for older age groups is fully recognised and vast prophylactic and therapeutic measures have been developed. The aim is to organise services to allow an old person to remain living in his own home. In Australia the care of the elderly is very much in the hands of the general practitioner, and there has been a gradual evolution of concepts of care. In Adelaide there is now an excellent domiciliary care service and the development of the Extra-Mural Hospital Services has been going on in New Zealand for a decade or more.

In most countries the need for an expanding and comprehensive community-based geriatric care team is becoming apparent and it is often in this area that future plans seem to be focused.

Notes

1. F. Adams, *The Genuine Works of Hippocrates* (Baltimore, Williams and Wilkins, 1939).
2. Brian Livesley, 'Historical Aspects of Ageing and Disease', *Modern Geriatrics*, vol.4, no.5 (1974), pp.204-12.
3. A translation of Galen's *Hygiene* by R.M. Green (Springfield, Thomas, 1951).
4. R. Bacon, *The Care of Old Age and Preservation of Youth*, translated by R. Browne (London, 1683).
5. I.L. Nascher, *Geriatrics: the Diseases of Old Age and their Treatment* (London, Pual, Trench and Trubner, 1919).
6. J.H. Sheldon, 'A History of British Geriatrics', *Modern Geriatrics*, vol.1, no.7 (1971), pp.457-64.
7. Lord Amulree, 'Welfare of the Elderly. An Historical Survey, *Modern Geriatrics*, vol.1, no.5 (1971), pp.330-5.
8. Ibid.
9. Laurie Lee, *Cider with Rosie* (Harmondsworth, Penguin Books. First published by the Hogarth Press, 1959).

10. J.H. Sheldon, 'The Role of the Aged in Modern Society', *British Medical Journal*, vol.1 (1950), pp.310-23.

11. J.H. Sheldon, 'Social Philosophy of Old Age', *Lancet*, vol.2 (1954), pp.151-5.

12. J. Williamson *et al.*, 'Old People at Home: Their Unreported Needs', *Lancet*, vol. 1 (1964), pp.1117-20.

Source Material and Further Reading

The articles by Lord Amulree, Brian Livesley and J.H. Sheldon quoted above.

J.C. Brocklehurst (ed.), *Geriatric Care in Advanced Societies* (Baltimore, University Park Press and Lancaster, MTP, 1975).

Fraser Brockington, *A Short History of Public Health* (London, Churchill Livingstone, 1966).

Ethel Shanas *et al.*, *Old People in Three Industrial Societies* (London, Routledge and Kegan Paul, 1968).

2 DEMOGRAPHIC CONSIDERATIONS

It is not the intention of this short chapter to give a comprehensive account of the changes that have occurred in the population structure of the UK during this century, nor to examine the reasons for these. Certain features are, however, so important to any consideration of the elderly in the community that a brief summary of the present position and possible future trends is necessary before proceeding to discuss contemporary problems.

J.A. Loraine, writing about world over-population, estimated that during 1976 more than 70 million people would be added to the planet.[1] No doubt this has in fact occurred and been repeated in 1977. The world's population by late 1975 had reached 4,000 million and is growing at the rate of 1.9 per cent per annum. The rate is expected to increase slightly during the next ten years and gradually slacken off by the year 2,000. Loraine quotes a UN estimate that the world total by the end of the century will be 6,250 million. However, within these overall figures, the developed countries show very different patterns of growth to poor countries. Fertility rates in the Third World remain high and it is likely that 90 per cent of the addition to the total population will take place in such countries.

The situation in developed countries such as the UK, is different. Here there is a change in the structure of the population so that there is an increasing proportion of elderly people within the overall total. There are now (1978) over 6.6 million people in England aged 65 and over, representing 14.3 per cent of the total population. If the UK as a whole is taken, these figures are even higher and it is expected that the total will continue to rise until 1990.

Even more striking, however, are the figures for over-75-year-old people. This is illustrated in Table 2.1, which shows an almost 20 per cent increase in their numbers in the past 15 years. The 1975 figures are provisional but nevertheless give a guide as to the trends. It is estimated that the numbers will rise by nearly one-third by 1995, to a figure just under three million. The number of people over 85 is expected to rise by an even higher percentage by 1995. This trend is a feature of most Western countries and is illustrated in Table 2.2. In general the proportion of persons over 65 years was at the level of about

Table 2.1: Population Trends for People Over 75 Years Old in England and Wales, 1961-75

Year	Population over 75 years old (England and Wales)
1961	1,987,700
1970	2,331,700
1975	2,489,000

Source: *Population Trends*, No.6 (Winter 1976), Table 15, p.51.

Table 2.2: Percentage of Population 65 Years Old and Over for Selected Countries, 1850 to 1970-5

Country	1850	1860	1880	1900	1920	1930	1940	1950	1970-5
France	6.5	6.9	8.1	8.2	9.1	9.4	–	11.8	13.6
United Kingdom	4.6	4.7	4.6	4.7	6.0	7.4	9.0	10.8	13.8
Sweden	4.8	5.2	5.9	8.4	8.4	9.2	9.4	10.3	14.5
Germany[a]	–	–	4.7	4.9	5.8	7.4	–	9.3	13.9
United States	–	–	–	4.1	5.7	5.4	6.9	8.1	10.3
Italy	–	4.2	5.1	6.2	6.8	–	7.4	–	10.9
Canada	–	–	–	5.1	4.8	5.6	6.7	7.8	8.3
Netherlands	4.8	4.9	5.5	6.0	5.9	6.2	7.0	7.7	10.4
Czechoslovakia	–	–	–	–	–	6.6	–	7.6	11.6

a. West Germany after 1950.

Source: United Nations, *Demographic Yearbook* (1974); United Nations, 'The Ageing of Populations', *Population Studies*, No.26 (1956). Reproduced from David Hobman, *The Social Challenge of Ageing* (London, Croom Helm, 1978).

4.5 per cent in the middle of the nineteenth century and even at the beginning of the twentieth century in certain countries, including the USA. The proportion has risen subsequently to between 10 per cent and 13 per cent in 1970. Thus, many people born at the end of the last century have survived to swell the numbers present today, yet life expectation among the old has not altered greatly. A 65-year-old man now lives on average only one year longer than such a man in 1841; a 65-year-old woman four and a half years longer.[2] The increase in the numbers of old people is of course due to the fact that more survive into old age.

A recent (1978) survey by Audrey Hunt reveals that after the age of 65 years, women outnumber men by more than 3 to 2.[3] She found that 52 per cent were married (nearly 75 per cent of men, but only 38 per cent of women); about 38 per cent were widowed (19 per cent of men and 50 per cent of women); 8 per cent were single and 2 per cent were divorced.

The number and relative proportions of elderly people in the community is growing at a startling rate. Particularly impressive and important is the rate at which the numbers of very old people is likely to grow until at least the beginning of the next century. These facts are bound to have a considerable impact on the planning and delivery of medical and social care for old people in the community.

Notes

1. J.A. Loraine, 'Overpopulation in 1976', *Update* vol. 12, no 9 (1976), pp.1047-9.
2. D.J. Jolley and Tom Arie, 'Organisation of Psycho-geriatric Services', *British Journal of Psychiatry*, vol.132 (1978), pp.1-11.
3. Audrey Hunt, *The Elderly at Home* (Office of Population Censuses and Surveys, Social Services Division) (London, HMSO, 1978).

3 AGEING AND HEALTH

Natural ageing is a subtle and little understood process. There is no point in time when a particular person becomes old and yet the difference between a 40-year-old man and an 80-year-old man is quite clear. Little is known about the mechanism of ageing, but insight into the natural history of old age is important when dealing with the diseases affecting old people. Aspects of ageing include not only physical and mental changes, but also social adaptations. These latter features will be discussed in the next chapter. Here, natural ageing and some of the theories of its causation will be described. Changes in bodily function will also be discussed together with the differing presentations and characteristics of illness in old age.

Normal Ageing

Old age and the wish to prolong life have long had a fascination. The Psalmist talked about the natural life span of three score years and ten and, ever since, men have desired to prolong this period of expected life Attaining this aim has so far proved impossible and the typical life span remains virtually the same. It is, however, being achieved by many more people. The chance of death increases exponentially with age and is influenced by two factors. The first is the ageing process itself and the second is disease, although it is sometimes difficult to distinguish between them.

When discussing life span, it is important to distinguish between conditions that hasten death in the form of disease, accident and various environmental factors, and those that are intrinsically part of the ageing process. The natural ageing process has been termed senescence and shows itself, as Comfort points out, as 'an increasing probability of death with increasing chronological age'.[4] This implies that changes take place in the body as time goes by, in the absence of recognised disease. Very often, however, the two processes of senescence and disease are going on side by side and one may well affect the other.

It is sometimes noticed that an old person just 'fades away' and here ageing must contribute to the eventual death. The time scale of ageing is also variable and it is well known that people can look much older than their chronological age would suggest, and similarly, many old people act and look much younger than their years. There is a saying that a man is as old as he feels and a woman as old as she looks and this perhaps hints at a different attitude to ageing shown by the two sexes. There is therefore often a difference between biological age and chronological age at any given point in a person's life, but this may alter as time progresses. It is also true that various organs age at different rates. These variations in ageing, not only in individuals but also of specific organs, make it difficult to study the factors influencing these processes. People of the same age group are often compared to determine features of actual ageing but these cross-sectional studies only confirm the variability of physiological response to the passage of time. Longitudinal studies of cohorts may reveal more information as to how vitality is lost. Comfort makes the point that if we kept the vitality throughout life that we had at the age of twelve, about half of us would still be here in 700 years' time. We should by dying off like radioactive atoms at a random rate and we would have no specific age beyond which we knew we were unlikely to live.

The Theories of Ageing

To study the ageing process the relatively new science of gerontology has emerged. The problems faced are highly complex and with experimentation being difficult, it is little wonder that scanty progress has been made in really understanding how and why organisms age. Nor have there been practical advances in increasing the life span. A dramatic improvement in the treatment of cardiovascular disease or cancer would not appreciably influence longevity. The life expectation of a 70-year-old person has not changed very much over recent years and a much more fundamental understanding of the problem of ageing is going to be necessary to achieve this; even with this understanding the objective may prove unattainable.

Many theories have been put forward as to the nature of ageing and some authors have actually proposed methods of prolonging the life span. One, for instance, involves the use of hormones in the hope that they might lead to extended youth. Ivor Felstein reviews many of the theories in his book *Living to be a Hundred.*[3] Early ideas such as the Hippocratic notion that old age was due to loss of body heat, or the anatomist Theodore Swann's view that vital life material was lost from somatic cells, were based on little evidence. But some later ideas, for instance that the environment played a part in affecting the rate of ageing, were at least based upon observations like the fact that social class can affect longevity. It has also been shown experimentally that radiation accelerates the process of ageing in laboratory animals and it is also known that over-feeding reduces the life span and in man there is a relationship between obesity and early death. Genetic influences can affect the likelihood of attaining extreme old age. There are long-lived families and Ivor Felstein mentions the Trevellyan family. Sir George Trevellyan died at the age of 90 and his son died at the age of 86. Sir Charles Trevellyan, who was Sir George's father, died at the age of 79. Many such pedigrees can be quoted so that genetics is obviously important. Different species have different life spans. Elephants live longer than mice. Is this because of different rates of cell division, or an inherently slower rate of ageing? It is likely that many factors are important and no single theory yet provides the answer. Perhaps gerontology has so far only been able to discard irrelevant theories and concentrate on defining the problem.

P.R.J. Burch,[4] in reviewing the main theories of ageing, divides them into four basic groups. The first is the programmed theory where senescence can be regarded as an inevitable stage in the sequence which begins at fertilisation and carries on through foetal life, birth, childhood, youth and on to maturity. As Burch points out, there are strong arguments against this view. The small spread in the age at which developing organisms attain each specific stage in development and the large spread in the age of onset of many conditions of ageing is one reason for rejecting the programmed theory. The appearance of an occasional grey hair before normal growth is finished is not exactly consistent with the theory. Comfort rejects the theory on other grounds and suggests that ageing is more likely to result from exhaustion of the programme.[5]

Secondly, there is the toxic theory which argues that poisonous substances accumulate in the organism and produce dysfunction and death. This theory also has faults and fails to account for the anatomical specificity of many age-dependent disorders.

The third group of theories can be described as wear and tear. Old age is likened to the wear of machines, and erosion of teeth is cited as an example, but it is impossible to apply this concept to such conditions as greying hair and arcus senilis.

The theories described so far are basically non-biological and are presumably, therefore, non-relevant. In an attempt to introduce biological principles, interest has centred on so-called error theories. Various theories fall into this category. Evidence is seen of ageing in various microscopic elements in the body. Extra-cellular connective tissue may show changes in structure and cells themselves may become defective. On a widespread scale, as with the loss or greying of hair, numerous cells develop defects more or less simultaneously. Burch considers that many of these macroscopic manifestations of ageing reflect a *relational* disturbance. That is, errors of synthesis of recognition proteins occur in one, or sometimes several, central growth control cells and the mutant products of their descendant cells attack target cells that bear complementary recognition proteins. The macrocytic consequences of the attack are observed in the *target* cells, which, in some instances, are distributed at many anatomical sites. This points to a controlling central factor. Two rather similar theories have been proposed along these lines, the auto-immune and the auto-aggressive. Both these theories are complex but basically the idea of the auto-immune theory is that mutations occur which produce immunological intolerance, resulting in self-impairment of cells and in certain disorders, death. The auto-aggressive theory is more fundamental and postulates mutation, not in the system that controls the normal immune response to particulate antigens but in the system that normally controls the size and growth of target tissues throughout the body.

Burch believes that ageing consists, in the main, of a constellation of specific age-dependent, auto-aggressive disorders that comprise both so-called physiological and pathological ageing. He distinguishes, however, the deterministic character of normal growth and development from the stochastic aspects of senescence which are initiated by random errors. Despite this fundamental distinction between deterministic and random processes, normal growth and senescence involve the same biological system.

No doubt in the end genes will be found to play a vital part. Richard Dawkins in his interesting book *The Selfish Gene* quotes Sir Peter Medawar's ingenious genetic theory of ageing. He postulates senile decay as being due to an accumulation in the gene pool of late-acting lethal or semi-lethal genes which have evolutionarily slipped through the net of natural selection because they are late-acting and so act beyond the normal reproducing period.[6]

These concepts are intriguing and obviously open the way to fundamental research, but it is clear that much work is still necessary before any practical solutions will be available to counteract the disorders of senescence and make it possible to achieve a longer life span.

Changes in Specific Systems in Old Age

It has been mentioned that cells and extra-cellular structures show changes with age and this is also true of the body itself and its various systems. The effects of natural senescence sometimes merge with the abnormal and it is important to recognise which is normal ageing and which is disease. Again, separate individuals and different organs vary in their rate of ageing. Sexual variations may be apparent but it is surprising as real old age advances, how men and women tend to look more alike.

Some physical changes are obvious. Height is reduced and the body becomes smaller due to loss of body weight. Very often there is thoracic kyphosis, particularly in women. The hair becomes grey and in both men and women it may be lost. Muscle power is reduced and the grip may be poor. Teeth are lost or at least the gum retracts giving the so-called 'long in the tooth' appearance. Control of body temperature is harder to achieve and old people easily become cold. Patterns of sleep may alter and night cramps occur with greater frequency. The voice changes and may grow thin, due to loss of elasticity of the laryngeal cartilage amd muscle.

Nervous System

Tendon and superficial reflexes are sometimes absent in old people. Anderson and Cowan in their Rutherglen series found abdominal reflexes absent in about 20 per cent of men and over 50 per cent of women.[5] Absent tendon reflexes were rare, but 5 per cent of healthy old men had no ankle reflexes. Sensory perception may be reduced in old age, particularly of the lower extremities and this applies especially to vibration sense. The overall pattern is for reduced sensory discrimination, particularly in the ability to perceive changes in temperature. As age advances, many nerve cells are lost or undergo degenerative changes, and there is some reduction in brain size.

Special Senses

The prevalence of deafness due to causes other than wax in the ear increases with age. Problems of maintaining balance become more common and not infrequently old people complain of tinnitus. Eyesight deteriorates as age advances and progressive long-sightedness starts by the mid-forties and continues into old age. The lens becomes increasingly opaque and less elastic. The pupillary reflex becomes slower and the diameter of the pupil decreases. Recovery from glare takes longer and there is a deterioration in dark adaption and colour vision. The sense of smell is also often diminished.

Digestive System

Deterioration of the digestive system is not particularly marked in old age. Both the liver and gall bladder appear to be little affected. Gastro-intestinal disturbances may be increased and there is a tendency towards constipation.

Respiratory System

Respiration efficiency is reduced along with the total lung volume. Oxygen diffusion in the lungs may be impaired and tissue utilisation is less efficient. The respiratory reserve capacity is reduced, probably due to impaired movement of the thoracic cage.

Cardiovascular System

Discussion is often heard about the normal range of blood pressure in old people. It has been hitherto accepted that readings of up to 200mm of mercury systolic and 100mm mercury diastolic are normal for men and even slightly higher readings are normal for women. Williams recorded the blood pressures of 270 unselected patients of over 75 years old (86 men and 184 women).[8] The mean of these readings in the various groups was calculated and these are shown in Table 3.1, with, for interest, the standard deviation. There has always been the feeling that blood pressure increases with age but these figures for the over-75-year-olds show that this is minimal and suggest that levels do not increase after 80 years. The levels in general were not particularly high and although they were higher in women, this sexual difference is probably minimal in old age. Survival seems to be more likely if the blood pressure is not high. These people probably represent a special group in the population with blood pressure stability. The findings would suggest that clinically it may be important to treat certainly patients over 75 with diastolic readings of over 105mm of mercury as this represents an abnormally high level. The reason for this is stroke prevention. More research needs doing as to whether the incidence would be reduced by such measures, but as stroke can leave such devastating after effects, prevention is important and should be attempted. Modern treatment with diuretics and beta blocking drugs is now easy and safe thus making feasible their use in old age.

The arteries in old age become thickened and hard, probably due to increased collagen in their walls, and calcification can occur. Veins

Table 3.1: Mean Level of Blood Pressure (with Standard Deviations) for Men and Women over 75 Years Old

Age Group	Mean Systolic and Standard Deviation in mm of Mercury	Mean Diastolic and Standard Deviation in mm of Mercury
a) Male		
75-79	155 ± 24.77	86 ± 10.9
80-84	162 ± 24.80	87 ± 11.53
85-89	171 ± 31.37	90 ± 12.14
90+	142 ± 26.39	81 ± 14.72
All ages 75+	159 ± 26.25	86 ± 11.28
b) Female		
75-79	163 ± 23.64	91 ± 8.84
80-84	158 ± 23.24	90 ± 13.63
85-89	159 ± 25.34	90 ± 12.65
90+	156 ± 11.40	88 ± 4.47
All ages 75+	160 ± 23.57	90 ± 11.48

Sample — 270 cases (86 men; 184 women).
Source: E.I. Williams, unpublished MD thesis, University of Manchester, 1973.

are less affected by ageing. Thoracic kyphosis often displaces the apex beat of the heart and this may also be masked by emphysema. As many as two-thirds of the patients over 70 have systolic ejection murmurs over the aortic area.

Haemoglobin

Williams estimated haemoglobin levels in 286 patients over 75 years of age.[9] Figure 3.1 shows a histogram of the distribution. The sexual difference between haemoglobin levels in ages up to 75 years has frequently been commented upon. From the study quoted, it would appear that this influence extends well beyond this age.

Endocrine System

It is difficult to assess the precise effect of ageing on the various endocrine glands. Thyroid function, for instance, is thought to decrease with age but there is no clear evidence of this. It is possible that the pituitary gland and adrenal gland are little affected. Secretion of sex hormones declines with age and this affects secondary sex features such as the breasts, which tend to atrophy. In men there is

Figure 3.1: Histogram of Haemoglobin Values in a Study of 297 People Over 75 Years Old (100% haemoglobin = 14.8g/100ml)

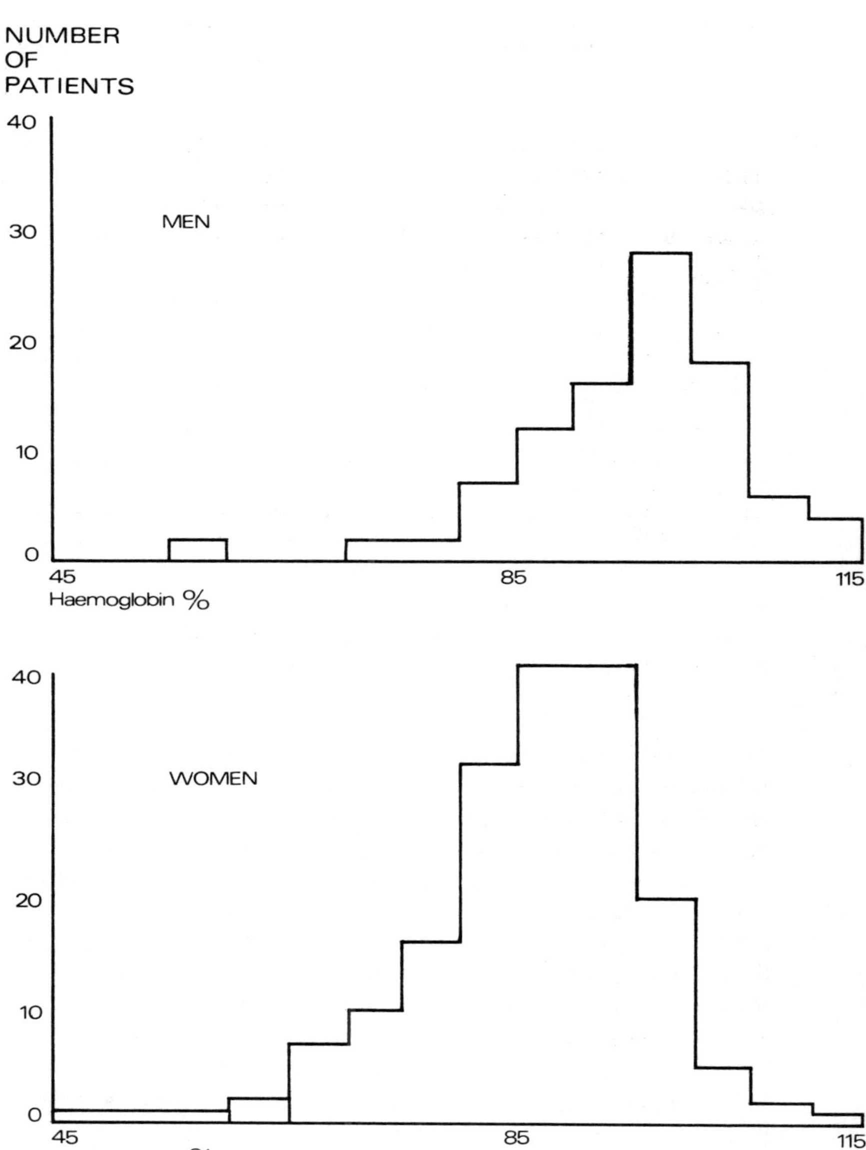

usually a progressive reduction in sexual function but recent evidence suggests that it is quite possible for sexual activity to survive well into old age.

Renal System

Changes do occur in renal function. There is evidence of a decline in glomerular filtration and renal blood flow. The acid/base balance is hard to maintain in old age.

The Skin

Changes in the skin are very noticeable. Environmental factors can affect these changes and prolonged exposure to sunlight can accelerate the process. Skin ageing also varies from person to person and it is possible that some hereditary influence is at work. The changes consist mainly of atrophy of the epidermis with an increase in pigmentation, and degenerative changes in the collagenous and elastic fibres of the dermis. Pigmented areas are seen more frequently and there is a high incidence of small papillomata. The skin looks thinner and shows more wrinkles and appears lax and dry. The subcutaneous fat may be reduced and the skin sometimes has a loose, hanging appearance. The nails grow at a slower rate and may be more brittle. There may be a reduction in sweat due to atrophy of the sweat glands. Hair follicles are reduced in density and the hair is markedly thinner, but curiously, rarely completely absent. Greying of the hair due to loss of melanin pigment is almost universal and the process can start at a very early age.

Psychological Aspects of Ageing

As well as physical changes, old age brings with it alteration in psychological outlook. This is variable but certain characteristics are recognisable and these probably arise from the cumulative effects of psychological adaptation to earlier stages in life. The pathway from early adulthood through middle adulthood to the pre-retirement phase of 60 to 65 usually consists of a complex series of events which contribute to psychological ageing. Sexual differences are apparent in this process. Women tend to live longer than men and psycho-social transitions are different for the two. Men may strive for independence, whereas women have tended to search for interdependence in marriage. Childbearing and rearing are of major importance to women and the subsequent adjustment to the eventual departure of children, as they too become independent, may be psychologically traumatic. Women may have to cope with their husband's eventual retirement and often widowhood as well. Social class differences are also present. Manual workers reach the summit of their working lives early, whereas professional people do not reach their maximum working capacity until much later. Successful psychological reassessment in middle age can have a bearing on attitudes in old age. Realisation that some ambitions will not be fulfilled and the adoption of realistic aims for the remaining available time are important in middle age and lead to a more contented old age. Many adjustments are necessary. Some men despair of their physical decline in middle age, whereas others are proud of their relative youth. Women, too, become more aware of their husband's health and think of the possibilities of his dying. They rehearse for widowhood, and sometimes plan along these lines. For instance, they may want to move into a smaller, more convenient house and look to their own financial security. These may of course be merely sensible arrangements taken in response to changing circumstances. Hopefully, adjustments will have been made to these problems before the major hurdle of retirement is reached. More will be said on this subject in Chapter 4, but there is the risk at this time that disengagement might occur and newly retired people might withdraw from the mainstream of life. Ideally, this should not happen and old people should retain their interest and activity, certainly in what has come to be known as 'young old age', from 65 to 75 years. Eventually, however, a stage is sometimes reached when an old person cannot cope with the demands of everyday living and becomes dependent on others. Some adapt to this, whereas others resent the whole concept of ageing and fear having to rely on others for help. People living by themselves, particularly if their personality was originally introverted, gradually withdraw from social contact and become isolated. When depression is present or physical neglect occurs these people can become quite desolate and may cut themselves off from help. Intelligence itself does not show much decline with ageing but the capacity to solve new problems deteriorates. Faced with the fear that they may no longer be able to solve problems, some old people may tend to become apathetic and often do not seek help even when this is readily available.

Changing Characteristics of Illness in Old Age

Probably the first thing to say about any illness in old age is that it needs to be looked at in physical, mental and social terms. The interdependence between the patient's environment, and his mental and physical state is often crucially important. Illness may often be due to a combination of problems and management must take into account all these factors. Pathology, of course, is more common in old age and there is a general increase in morbidity. Some diseases are age-related. Generalised arteriosclerosis and osteoporosis are two examples. Not surprisingly, multiple disability is so common as to be almost the rule. Thomas, in running a clinic for the elderly, found that more than 80 per cent of his group had multiple disability and numerous other surveys have supported this finding.[10] Many of the conditions found are degenerative in type but some are amenable to treatment. Many are minor, but the problem is that the presence of several of these can set up a vicious circle, resulting in a reduction in a patient's functional capacity, and severe disablement ensues. An example of conditions interacting in this way is obesity affecting osteoarthritic knees and possible cardiac impairment. The presence of anaemia may also adversely affect the course of many conditions.

Multiple symptomatology is also a common finding. Elderly patients can have many complaints and will usually admit to many more on direct questioning. Some symptoms impair health more than others. In the author's survey of over-75-year-olds dizziness or giddiness was a common symptom occurring more frequently in patients of poor effective health.[11] Forgetfulness is another distressing symptom of old age. Symptoms must also be interpreted differently in old age. Ferguson Anderson, for instance, attaches the same significance to confusion in an old person as to convulsions in a baby, that is, it might be produced by a number of causes, including anything which increases the temperature.[12] Old people may have a different threshold of pain and may complain of it less frequently. They also do not seem to appreciate thirst as acutely. Temperature changes may also not be noticed. Physical signs of illness in the aged need assessing differently. The changes already described which occur with natural ageing, influence, for instance, the measurement of heart size and position.

Illnesses in old age may have unusual clinical presentations. Infections often progress insidiously and may only be discovered at an advanced stage. In some infections the temperature does not necessarily always rise and the white cells count remains normal. Tuberculosis sometimes presents as no more than general weakness and tiredness. Non-specific failure to thrive can be due to bacteraemia. Presentation of both thyroid over- and underactivity may be very atypical in old age. R.A. Griffiths, in an excellent article on thyroid disease of the elderly, quotes seven possible ways hidden hyperthyroidism may present.[13] These he lists as:

1. unexplained heart failure with atrial fibrillation;
2. loss of weight and anorexia;
3. malabsorption, diarrhoea or constipation;
4. acute or chronic muscular weakness;
5. fits, chorea, exacerbation of Parkinsonian tremor;
6. abnormal psychiatric states;
7. apathetic hyper-thyroidism. Patients 'old for their age'; showing ptosis, cardiac failure and atrial dysrhythmia, loss of weight, muscle wasting and cool, dry pigmented skin.

He also points out that the insidious onset of myxoedema makes the diagnosis difficult even although the presentation is typical.

Heart disease too, has various presentations in old age. Angina is relatively uncommon; myocardial infarction occurs but is difficult to diagnose clinically as pain only occurs in about a quarter of the cases and the attack may be asymptomatic.[14] Confusion and restlessness are usually present in acute infarction and most forms of heart failure. Diabetes mellitus can also present atypically and may first be noticed as bed-wetting or incontinence. An illness in old age can be complicated by such factors as hypothermia, sensitivity to drugs and sub-nutrition. Dehydration easily occurs and can cloud the clinical picture.

Unreported Need

In the 1950s it became apparent to geriatricians that many patients were being referred too late in their illness for any effective action to be taken. It was felt that more could have been done if the patients themselves had sought attention at an earlier stage. Surveys were undertaken to study the health of old people in the community, an early one being that of Hobson and Pemberton in Sheffield.[15] They describe how a good deal of previously undiagnosed illness was discovered and although some was minor and of little significance, a small number of serious, treatable conditions were encountered. These included diabetes, myxoedema, rodent ulcer and scurvy.

Williamson *et al.*, working in Edinburgh, again noted the striking and distressing feature of patients being often admitted to a geriatric unit in a very advanced stage of disease.[16] They were impressed by the fact that this had been unknown to the family doctor, and carried out a survey on a random sample of persons aged 65 and over who were on the list of three general practitioners in Edinburgh. A total of 200 people were examined. There were 170 disabilities unknown to the general practitioner amongst men, and 221 disabilities unknown to the general practitioner amongst women. This type of result has been confirmed by subsequent surveys. Williams examined 297 patients over 75 years of age and found many previously unreported conditions and social needs.[17] He found seven malignant conditions, 28 patients with heart failure, five with diabetes and one with myxoedema. A high incidence of nutritional anaemia was detected. Many minor conditions were also found and treatment was necessary for 184 of the patients. Forty-three were referred to outpatient clinics and 40 to the local social service department. Nearly 50 people required chiropody treatment. Currie *et al.*, in a study of patients aged 70 to 72, quote an incidence of 20.5 per cent of disability which was unknown to the doctor.[18] He supports the view that the value of finding these unreported conditions is that, although many may be minor, if untreated, they limited the old person's ability to cope with everyday life. Hay in a survey with a high response rate, found pathological conditions of which no one was aware in one in four of his patients.[19]

However, not all surveys have discovered that there has been much unreported need. Irwin[20] from Finhagey found few cases of established organic disease which were unknown to the doctor. He thought this was perhaps due to good doctor/patient relationships and the fact that Finhagey is a small, well-defined community. Evans *et al.*, in a survey of their country practice, found little, if any, in the way of serious problems which were unknown to the doctors.[21] The survey did have a fairly low response rate and the practice was a rural one. It is probable that in rural areas or small practices the doctors know personally a higher proportion of their old patients. Jones defines doctor ignorance rates as the proportion of cases known to the general practitioner in comparison to those found by screening and quotes this as varying between 30 per cent and 60 per cent.[22] Low rates seem to be found in rural areas and Jones finds it tempting to extend Tudor Hart's inverse care law to geriatric screening, namely that the quantity of unmet need discovered at geriatric screening is inversely proportional to the care that patients normally receive.

It seems from this type of evidence that old people cannot tell when they are unwell. This means that disease is not detected at an early stage and, as Ferguson Anderson puts it, 'there is an iceberg of unreported illness amongst the old people in the community.' Why should this be so? Several reasons have been advanced. There is a general apathy and lack of initiative in old people and they have the idea that such conditions as breathlessness and ankle swelling are not due to illness but are an integral part of old age. Old people may find it difficult to attend the doctor's surgery because of lack of transport or inconvenient hours; but perhaps it is more a fear of what might happen when they arrive and many have an aversion to being admitted to hospital or undergoing investigation. Again, they may feel that they do not want to trouble the doctor with conditions they think are basically untreatable. It seems a problem primarily of urban society and it is interesting to contemplate why this should be. Perhaps isolation is more common in towns than in the country.

What are the sorts of disability which are unreported and unknown to the doctor? Although in all surveys serious conditions such as malignant disease, heart failure and diabetes were found, many of the problems were relatively minor. These would include such conditions as hallux valgus, toe-nail deformity, varicose veins, skin lesions, inguinal hernia, osteoarthritis and Dupuytren's contracture. In women various conditions of the genito-urinary system, like vulvo-vaginitis, cervical polyp, prolapse, urethral caruncle and urinary infections were found. Perhaps this is due to the intimate nature of the symptoms and old ladies' reluctance to discuss such 'private problems'. In men, hydrocele and prostatic symptoms were often unreported for the same reason. Eye and ear conditions also figure largely in the findings, including deafness caused by the infinitely treatable wax in the ear. Many mental conditions, too, tended to be unreported.

Some old people refuse to co-operate in screening exercises and they have been the subject of special study. Akhtar shows that the physical and mental health of uncooperative patients was little different from others and other studies have confirmed this.[23] In the author's survey, 45 patients were originally unwilling to take part and subsequently 41 of these were visited.[24] A high proportion of these patients lived alone. Many might have accepted the invitation to attend had more reassurance as to its purpose been given. Over two-thirds of them were, however, in good health and they generally resembled the acceptor patients in conditions found.

Effective Health

Many old people have multiple disability, but despite this, it is obvious to anyone working with them that they are able to cope and that their ability to live a normal life is not impaired. Functional capacity is therefore more important than the presence of disease. For this reason, the concept of effective health has been introduced. Hobson and Pemberton were the first to recognise this and although they did not enumerate pathological conditions, they did attempt to assess the effective health of the group.[25]

The author in his 1972 survey attempted to determine the effective health of 297 patients over 75 years old.[26] They divided into three groups as defined below.

1. Patients who were able to do their own cooking, housework and shopping; had a cheerful and normal mental state and no incapacitating illness.
2. Patients whose movements were restricted, often housefast, unable to do their own shopping, but were able to cook and do some housework. Mental deterioration may have been present but they were coping with the situation. These patients often had illnesses but were able to manage to deal with their problems.
3. These were usually bedfast patients. They were unable to cook, do their housework or shopping. There was often general restriction of movements. They may have had mental deterioration or incapacitating illness.

Patients did not necessarily need to have each of the factors mentioned to be included in a particular group. Thus, if a patient was suffering from severe debilitating illness but not bedfast, he was nevertheless put into group 3. The resulting grouping was as follows:

group 1	176 patients	60 per cent
group 2	108 patients	36 per cent
group 3	13 patients	4 per cent

A reasonable percentage of people were therefore in good effective health and obviously coping well in the community. Those in poorer effective health were more vulnerable and in overall terms, these were people who might have benefited from some sheltered care. It is difficult, however, to generalise. Some, even in poor effective health, were well adapted to the environment in which they were living and although they would have been unable to cope for themselves, had help enough to produce an equilibrium of care. Each old person must be considered as an individual in assessing his circumstances and needs. This means seeing him as a member of society. This aspect will be discussed in the next chapter.

Notes

1. Psalm 90, verse 10.
2. A. Comfort, *Ageing. The Biology of Senescence* (London, Routledge and Kegan Paul, 1964).
3. Ivor Felstein, *Living to be a Hundred. A Study of Old Age* (Newton Abbott, David and Charles, 1973).
4. P.J.R. Burch, 'The Biological Nature of Ageing', *Symposia of Geriatric Medicine*, vol.3 (West Midlands Institute of Geriatric Medicine and Gerontology, 1974).
5. Comfort, *Ageing.*
6. Richard Dawkins, *The Selfish Gene* (London, Oxford University Press, 1976).
7. W. Ferguson Anderson, *Practical Management of the Elderly* (Oxford and Edinburgh, Blackwell Scientific Publications, 1967), p.220.
8. E.I. Williams, unpublished MD thesis, Manchester University, 1973.
9. E.I. Williams *et al.*, 'Sociomedical Study of Patients over 75 in General Practice', *British Medical Journal*, vol.2 (1972), pp.445-8.
10. P. Thomas, 'Experience of Two Preventative Clinics for the Elderly', *British Medical Journal*, vol.2 (1968), pp.357-60.
11. Williams, MD thesis.
12. Anderson, *Practical Management.*
13. R.A. Griffiths, 'Thyroid Disease in the Elderly', *Update* vol. 12, no. 4 (1976), p.343.
14. Mario Impalomini, 'Heart Disease in Old Age', *Update*, Part 1 vol. 8, no. 10 (1974), p.1367, Part 2 vol. 8, no. 11 (1974), p.1539.
15. W. Hobson and J. Pemberton, 'The Health of the Elderly at Home', *British Medical Journal*, vol.1 (1956), pp.587-93.
16. J. Williamson *et al.*, 'Old People at Home: Their Unreported Needs', *Lancet*, 23 May 1964, pp.1117-20.
17. Williams *et al.*, 'Sociomedical Study of Patients over 75'.
18. G. Currie *et al.*, 'Medical and Social Screening of Patients aged 70 to 72 by an Urban General Practice Health Team', *British Medical Journal*, vol.2 (1974), pp.108-11.
19. E.H. Hay, 'A Geriatric Survey in General Practice', *Practitioner*, no.216 (April 1976), pp.443-7.
20. W.G. Irwin, 'Geriatric Practice in the Health Centre', *Modern Geriatrics* vol. 1, no. 4 (1971), pp.265-6.
21. S.M. Evans *et al.*, 'Growing Old. A Country Practice Survey', *Journal of the Royal College of General Practitioners*, vol.20, no.100 (1970), pp.278-84.
22. R.V.H. Jones, 'Recognition of Geriatric Problems in General Practice', *Update*, vol.13, no.7 (1976), p.643.
23. A.J. Akhtar, 'REfusal to Participate in a Survey of the Elderly', *Gerontologia Clinica*, vol.14 (1972), pp.205-11.
24. Williams *et al.*, 'Sociomedical Study of Patients over 75'.
25. Hobson and Pemberton, 'The Health of the Elderly at Home'.
26. Williams *et al.*, 'Sociomedical Study of Patients over 75'.

4 OLD PEOPLE IN SOCIETY

In this chapter the social background and material circumstances of old people will be described. Ageing is a social as well as a physical process and the passage of time usually brings with it altered domestic circumstances. Old people are also part of the community itself and are subject to any social changes which are occurring within it. Although there has been a supposition that the old may be particularly vulnerable to these changes, it is possible that there have been, until recently, protective mechanisms which have averted the worst of the problems which might have affected old people. These mechanisms rested in the family but there are now hints that they may be weakening. The extent to which family support for old people is changing can be seen by comparing the classic Townsend survey in 1962, *The Aged in the Welfare State*,[1] and a recently published survey by Audrey Hunt, *The Elderly at Home.*[2] It would appear that the availability of relatives has diminished since 1962, for not only are more elderly people living alone, but the number with no living relatives (5 per cent in *Elderly at Home* compared with 3 per cent in *Aged in the Welfare State*) is also increasing. Fewer old people also see relatives regularly. Eighty-four per cent of the earlier sample had seen a relative in the past week, compared with 71 per cent of the later sample, who either visited or were visited by a relative about once a week.[3] There are of course other means of contact, such as the telephone, and perhaps amongst middle class people this is used more frequently.

However, the general picture of old people in society is not too discouraging. Audrey Hunt's survey, which incidentally was of persons aged 65 years and over, found evidence that physical old age in the sense that it is generally understood does not begin at 65 for the great majority of people. Most between the ages of 65 and 74 were able to go out without assistance, were basically in reasonable health, and enjoyed hobbies, interests and social contacts. The housing conditions and amenities were not greatly inferior to those of younger people. Nevertheless, as age advances, changes do occur. In the 75-84 age group, a moderate decline was found in mobility, health and the ability to perform personal and domestic tasks. In other things there was a much sharper decline, as for instance in social contacts outside the home (except for centres for the elderly) and in having hobbies and interests.

Also the standards of housing and amenities were, on average, lower. Among those over 85, virtually all these trends were accentuated although there were still many who enjoyed good health and a full social life. As would be expected, advancing old age brought with it problems with health, social contact and living conditions, but as Audrey Hunt points out, the old are not a homogeneous group, but differ in their needs. She makes the point that people born before 1911 had lived through two world wars and the intense depression of the thirties. The oldest had retired or become widowed not very long after the 1939-45 War. It is not surprising, therefore, that the old of today generally have lower expectations than other age groups.

Everyone needs the basic requirements of living, including shelter (housing), food, clothes, warmth, toileting facilities, cleanliness and safety. There is also the necessity for privacy, which old people in particular find important. Over and above these, most people also require interest to gain personal satisfaction and enjoy a reasonable standard of life. The elderly are no exception. Meeting these requirements means being able to undertake certain personal tasks (see Table 4.1) and also certain domestic tasks (see Table 4.2). These will be discussed more fully in Chapter 6 but apart from the physical ability of being able to perform them, certain basic facilities are also necessary. These will be described in this chapter and will involve an examination of housing possibilities, economic situations, transport,

Table 4.1: Examples of Personal Tasks

1. Cutting toe-nails
2. Climbing stairs
3. Using public transport
4. Bathing
5. Getting out of doors
6. Getting around house
7. Getting in and out of bed
8. Getting to lavatory
9. Shaving/combing hair
10. Washing
11. Feeding yourself

Source: A Barlow and D. Matthews, 'Need for and Receipt of Domiciliary Social Services amongst the Elderly', unpublished DHSS Statistical Paper, March 1978. 1978.

Table 4.2: Examples of Domestic Tasks

1. Decorating
2. Carrying out minor repairs
3. Cleaning windows outside
4. Climbing stairs
5. Washing the paintwork
6. Cleaning windows inside
7. Washing floors
8. Sewing
9. Washing clothes
10. Sweeping floors
11. Unscrewing jars
12. Cooking
13. Using frying pan
14. Making a cup of tea

Source: Barlow and Matthews, 'Need for and Receipt of Domiciliary Social Services'.

social contact and interests and hobbies.

About one-fifth of the elderly population live in rural districts and one-third in major conurbations. In some popular retirement areas, over one-third of the population is elderly and some resorts face the prospect that during the next decade more than half their residents will be pensioners.[4] Little information is available about the type of housing old people inhabit (whether they live in houses, flats or tenements) and also their distribution within the community. Certain other information is, however, well documented and will now be discussed.

Old People Living Alone

Estimates of the number of old people living alone vary, but it is probably increasing, and is higher in the older age groups. Rosamund Gruer in her study *The Needs of the Elderly in the Scottish Borders* found 33 per cent living alone.[5] From Table 4.3 it can be seen that Audrey Hunt's survey found 29.6 per cent of persons living alone, with a very clear increase in the relative numbers as age advances. There is also a preponderance of women.

The definition of living alone has varied and it is difficult to compare

Table 4.3: Type of Household in which Elderly People Live (by Age within Sex of Elderly Persons)

	Men and Women				Men				Women			
	Grand Total	Age 65-74	75-84	85+	All Men	Age 65-74	75-84	85+	All Women	Age 65-74	75-84	85+
All elderly persons (weighted)	3,869	2,571	1,089	209	1,540	1,101	384	55	2,329	1,470	705	254
(unweighted figures)	2,622	1,354	1,063	205	994	565	375	54	1,628	789	688	151
Type of Household	%	%	%	%	%	%	%	%	%	%	%	%
1. One elderly person alone	29.6	25.0	37.4	44.0	15.6	13.6	19.8	27.3	38.8	33.6	47.1	50.0
2. One elderly person with non-elderly spouse only	7.4	10.4	1.7	–	15.8	20.5	4.4	–	1.9	2.9	0.3	–
3. One elderly person with next generation only	6.7	4.3	10.6	17.2	2.9	2.0	4.2	10.9	9.3	6.0	14.0	19.5
4. One elderly person, non-elderly spouse and next generation	1.7	2.4	0.3	–	4.2	5.6	0.8	–	–	–	–	–
5. One elderly person with others	5.9	5.6	6.4	7.7	4.7	4.2	6.0	7.2	6.7	6.7	6.7	7.7
6. Elderly married couple only	36.7	40.2	33.1	11.5	46.0	43.5	55.5	30.9	30.4	37.8	20.9	4.5
7. Elderly siblings only	2.8	2.3	3.9	2.9	1.0	0.8	1.0	5.5	4.0	3.4	5.5	1.9
8. Elderly married couple with next generation only	4.1	5.1	2.3	1.4	5.1	5.5	4.2	3.6	3.4	4.7	1.3	0.6
9. Other combinations of two or more elderly persons with others	5.1	4.7	4.2	15.3	4.5	4.2	4.2	14.5	5.5	5.0	4.3	15.6
Total	100.0	100.0	100.0	100.0	100.0	100.0	100.0	100.0	100.0	100.0	100.0	100.0

Source: A. Hunt, 'The Elderly at Home', Office of Population Censuses and Surveys (Social Survey Division) (London, HMSO, 1978), Table 4.6.1.

different studies. It may not imply being socially isolated and without contact with neighbours and relatives. In fact, the reverse is often true, particularly if an old person has lived in the same area for most of his or her life. Many old people live alone by choice, and although acceptance of a measure of loneliness is necessary, they nevertheless enjoy an active social life. A distinction therefore has to be made between those living alone and the section within this main group who might be called 'isolates'. These are people who do not have any contact with friends or relatives and may often be found in a miserable and neglected state. The main members of this group are the unmarried and those who never had children. There is also more risk of elderly persons being socially isolated if they had sons and not daughters. Young men are more easily drawn into their wives' families and may lose contact with their own parents. Fathers tend to have weaker ties with children and old men living alone are very liable to have no contact with their offspring. This may however be a class-related phenomenon, and middle-class sons do tend to have stronger ties with their fathers.

Loneliness, on the other hand, is a different type of experience and this may happen even if an old person is living with a large family. By contrast, some who live in extreme isolation maintain that they are never lonely, and obviously have inner resources to aid them. This is helped by the previous life-style and if letter-writing and telephone communication have been the habit, communications are maintained. There are, however, special situations which help to produce social isolation and loneliness and these will be discussed in the chapter on social vulnerability. People living alone are subject to many hazards. In the author's survey, for instance, most of those who had inadequate diets lived by themselves and many of these were anaemic.[6]

Family Structure of Those Not Living Alone

The most recent information as to the family structure of old people not living alone is given by Audrey Hunt, and can be seen in Table 4.3. As expected, husband and wife living together in a one-generation household is the most common pattern. It might be presumed that these couples managed their own domestic affairs, but there is evidence from other surveys (Rosamund Gruer) to suggest that much help is also usually forthcoming from relatives and friends in these circumstances and few of these old people were obliged to be self-sufficient. The Rosamund Gruer survey was undertaken in the Scottish Borders and the high level of help available might reflect the basically rural character of the region. The reason for living in a one-generation household was sometimes because the old couple had no children and when this was the case, there was similar evidence that domestic co-operation occurred between brothers and sisters of the same generation. The level of support which two old people, whether married or siblings, can give to each other, is quite remarkable and despite frailty, they manage to cope with their own domestic problems.

A sizeable minority of old people live in a two-generation home. This is where a house is shared with children, either married or unmarried, and sometimes another generation is involved, when there are grandchildren. Two-generation households sometimes require considerable role adjustment by the members, particularly the two women. When the shared house is the original family home, the mother's authority is usually maintained, especially over a daughter-in-law, but friction can easily occur and when the older woman becomes frail, there is danger of her becoming a subordinate housekeeper. Harmony can only be preserved by responsibilities being carefully defined. This is one reason why people prefer to live alone. It is easier when unmarried children live with old parents, because the old mother retains her role, but this can be affected by her state of health. This is particularly so when an old couple live with their son and daughter-in-law. It is easier for an old person to reciprocate services when there are grandchildren to look after and baby-sitting is necessary. The incidence of three-generation households is probably diminishing and this may be due to the desire of young people to create an independent home away from their parents, and their increasing economic ability to do so. Old people also may want to live alone and value their privacy – especially when the house, as is becoming more likely, is small.

Tenure of Accommodation

Surveys of the tenure of accommodation occupied by old people have often been undertaken. The recent studies by Audrey Hunt are typical and the results are shown in Table 4.4.[7] The figures need a little explanation because the actual numbers are increased by weighting. This was because relatively more people over 75 years old were interviewed in order to obtain sufficient numbers for detailed analysis and weighting is a device to restore proportions. The head of the household is the person who owns or is responsible for the rent, provided that he or she is present in the household and provided she is not a married woman, where a husband is present. In the latter case, her husband is the head of the household. A distinction is later made between an elderly head and a younger head. The first means a person

Table 4.4. Tenure of Dwelling (by Sex, Age, Marital Status of Head of Household, Type of Household, Region and Population Density)

	Elderly HOH Weighted	Unweighted figures	Tenure					
			Owned			Rented		Rent free
			Outright	Mortgage	Not answered	Council	Private	
Households with elderly heads	(2,705)	(1,811)	45.2	2.6	0.7	31.1	17.1	3.3
Sex of HOH[a]								
Man	(1,509)	(956)%	47.2	3.6	0.8	29.8	15.8	2.7
Woman	(1,196)	(855)%	42.7	1.3	0.6	32.8	18.6	4.0
Age of HOH								
64 and under	(54)	(29)%	37.0	9.3	—	37.0	9.3	7.4
65-74	(1,718)	(865)%	46.3	3.0	0.6	30.8	16.5	2.8
75-84	(789)	(776)%	44.4	1.6	1.0	30.8	18.6	3.5
85 and over	(144)	(141)%	41.0	—	0.7	34.7	18.8	4.9
Type of household								
Elderly person on own	(1,144)	(809)%	38.7	1.1	0.3	35.1	19.6	5.1
Elderly couple only	(996)	(626)%	49.8	2.8	0.9	28.6	15.6	2.3
Elderly siblings only	(54)	(41)%	64.8	—	3.7	7.4	22.2	1.9
One elderly with others	(360)	(228)%	47.2	5.6	0.3	31.1	14.7	1.2
More than one with others	(151)	(107)%	53.0	6.0	2.0	25.8	11.9	1.3
Marital status of HOH								
Married	(1,190)	(741)%	48.9	3.4	0.9	29.2	15.4	2.0
Widowed	(1,239)	(893)%	41.6	1.8	0.5	34.8	17.7	3.6
Single	(216)	(144)%	46.8	1.4	0.9	24.5	21.3	5.1
Divorced etc.	(60)	(33)%	41.7	6.7	—	16.7	23.3	11.6
Standard region								
North	(172)	(112)%	34.3	1.2	—	52.9	8.7	2.9
Yorkshire and Humberside	(268)	(188)%	38.8	2.2	—	41.4	15.3	2.3
North-West	(379)	(258)%	46.7	2.4	—	31.7	16.9	2.4
E. Midlands and E. Anglia	(377)	(253)%	51.5	2.9	—	30.0	13.5	2.1
W. Midlands	(276)	(182)%	46.4	1.8	—	33.0	17.4	1.4
Greater London	(350)	(230)%	33.7	3.7	2.6	24.9	32.9	2.3
South-East and South-West	(571)	(381)%	45.4	1.6	0.9	31.5	14.4	6.4
'Retirement areas'	(312)	(207)%	59.3	4.8	1.6	15.7	14.7	3.8
Population density								
Greater London	(350)	(230)%	33.7	3.7	2.6	24.9	32.9	2.3
Metropolitan counties	(692)	(470)%	41.2	1.9	—	39.3	16.3	1.2
Non-metropolitan counties:								
high	(345)	(231)%	47.0	4.1	0.9	28.7	18.6	0.9
medium	(377)	(246)%	48.3	4.0	—	28.9	14.1	4.8
low	(941)	(634)%	50.7	1.6	0.7	29.2	12.4	5.3

a. HOH = Head of household.

Source: Hunt, 'The Elderly at Home'.

aged 65 or over or a head aged less than 65 who is the husband of a woman aged 65 or over. The second means a person aged less than 65 who is not the husband of a woman aged 65 or over.

The study was confined to the elderly at home and not in institutions. About 6 per cent of the elderly persons can be expected to be in institutions, the relative percentage rising with age. There are striking regional differences between the levels of home ownership and council renting, as can be seen from Table 4.4.

Household Amenities

The most recent survey of the household state of old people is again that of Audrey Hunt. She gives a good account of the present level of amenity.

According to interviewers' assessments nearly 70 per cent of dwellings occupied by households with elderly heads were in good condition both internally and externally. The standards were markedly below average among households with heads aged 85 and over. Lower standards were also found amongst private tenants and in Greater London.

Overcrowding in terms of persons per room was not a problem for most households with elderly heads, but amongst households with younger heads it appears that in some cases the amount of living space was less than satisfactory. This indicates that there may be problems for some younger people in having elderly relatives living with them.

Virtually all households had a separate unshared kitchen; the only exception being a small group who live rent-free, where there is an increased incidence of sharing. Ninety per cent of households with an elderly head had a bathroom compared with 95 per cent of households with a younger head. Some groups were markedly below the average for this amenity and they included private tenants, those in Greater London, and those living rent-free. Twelve per cent of households with an elderly head had an outside toilet only. Ninety-two per cent of households with an elderly head and 99 per cent of those with a younger head had a hot water supply. Virtually all households had electricity and over two-thirds had mains gas. Where there was a choice of fuels for cooking, that which was cheaper at the time of the survey (gas) was more likely to be used. Thirty per cent of bedrooms occupied by the elderly were unheated. In the North-West region, the West Midlands region and amongst private tenants, this was higher and up to 40 per cent of the bedrooms were unheated. Three per cent of households had no heating in the living-room and just over half of all

Table 4.5 (a): Household Amenities and Possessions of Persons Aged 65 and Over

	Households with Elderly Heads (per cent)	Households with Young Heads (per cent)
Separate bathroom	90	95
Outside toilet only	12	7
Hot water supply	92	99
Electricity supply	100	100
Telephone	44	72
Car	28	73
Washing machine	53	83
Refrigerator	75	95

Source: Hunt, 'The Elderly at Home'.

Table 4.5 (b): Percentage of Rooms Occupied by Persons Aged 65 and Over Which are Heated (per cent)

	Per cent
Bedroom	70
Living room	97
Halls and passages	50
Bathroom	63
Lavatory	40
Kitchen	52

Source: Hunt, 'The Elderly at Home'.

households did not heat halls or passages. Thirty-seven per cent did not heat the bathroom; 60 per cent did not heat the lavatory and 48 per cent had no additional heating in the kitchen. In all cases, households with younger heads had on average better provisions for heating, while private tenants and households where the head was 85 or over had worse provisions. Forty per cent of households used solid fuels. About 10 per cent of all elderly householders had to go more than 10 feet outside in order to fetch solid fuel.

Households with elderly heads were much less likely than those with younger heads to own items of domestic equipment which are taken for granted by many younger people. Forty-four per cent of all households had a telephone but only 35 per cent of the elderly living alone, and 35 per cent of households with heads aged 85 or over, had one.

Income Level

Audrey Hunt's survey, which was carried out in January and February 1976, found that there was a marked decline in income level with age. Half the married couples living on their own had an income level of less than £1,500 per year and 68 per cent of non-married people living alone had an income of less than £1,000 per year. Sixty-one per cent of non-married people with incomes of less than £1,000 lived alone. Fourteen per cent of married couples and 28 per cent of non-married persons were solely dependent on the state retirement pension and/or supplementary benefits. Fifty-one per cent of husbands compared with 6 per cent of wives had pensions from previous employers. Low income was associated with lack of assets or only very small assets. In addition to the 12 per cent who received Supplementary Benefits, 11 per cent of married couples had an income of less than £1,500 a year, together with assets of less than £300. Among non-married persons, 31 per cent of the total received Supplementary Benefits and a further 13 per cent had incomes of less than £750 per year, together with assets of less than £300.

Transport

According to Audrey Hunt, two-thirds of elderly people live in households with no car. Nine-tenths of those living alone, compared with two-fifths of those living with younger people, have no access to a car. All elderly people in households with a car use it, whether they drive or not. About one-third of those without cars are taken out at least once a fortnight by people outside the household. Visiting, shopping, pleasure trips, holidays and medical visits are the main purposes for which cars are used. The level of car ownership and use is much lower in Greater London than elsewhere. Two-thirds of elderly people live in areas where there are special transport facilities for the elderly. There are wide differences between areas, the best-off being Greater London, and the worst-off, the retirement areas. Four-fifths of elderly persons are within ten minutes' walk of the nearest public transport. Over half are able to walk to the nearest chemist's shop. Nine-tenths of those who go to pubs walk there. Three-quarters walk to the nearest Post Office. The doctor's surgery is the only one of the listed amenities to which the majority require some means of transport and for which a majority take more than ten minutes' walk over the journey. As might be expected, the use of transport increases with age.

Interests and Hobbies

Audrey Hunt makes comments on the hobbies and attitudes of old people to life. She found that, taken overall, the evidence was that elderly people were as likely as others to want to have hobbies and interests. There was, however, a very marked falling off with increasing age in the proportion who kept pets, who participated in voluntary organisations, who had individual hobbies and interests or who had any hobbies at all. The bedfast and housebound were undoubtedly least able to maintain activities and were not unexpectedly much less contented, in the sense that they had nothing to enjoy, than other groups. The most contented group of all were the elderly workers. Ill-health was the principal thing disliked, followed by loneliness. Financial difficulty was mentioned by comparatively few, but when asked for suggestions to help elderly people, financial matters predominated. However, a higher proportion wanted volunteers to chat to or for company than any other single form of help.

Social Contacts

Audrey Hunt also found that the majority of elderly people do not go to any kind of social centre and, taking social contacts with people outside the household as a whole, the housebound and bedfast particularly are the most severely isolated. Other groups who are relatively badly off in this respect are those aged 85 and over, and divorced persons.

Housefast People

In the same study it was found that 0.3 per cent of people were permanently bedfast and a further 4.2 per cent permanently confined to the dwelling. The figures are lower than were found in earlier surveys and as Audrey Hunt says, this may be due to slight differences in definition and to the increase in car ownership. Other surveys, particularly those confined to older age groups, have found an incidence of housefast people as high as 20 per cent. Undoubtedly, the proportion increases with age, and it is relatively more common in women. Perhaps the greatest cause for concern found by Audrey Hunt was that one-quarter of those unable to go out, even with assistance, lived on their own and were therefore dependent on outsiders for everything that needed to be brought from outside.

Family Care

The word family needs defining because of its different meanings. A nuclear family refers usually to one which is living in the same household, whereas an extended family would involve uncles, aunts and cousins and is normally three generations. Between these there is a variety of relationships but what is meant by a family, certainly as a source of help by the caring professions, is a three-generation unit.

How do families usually care for their elderly members? A few tentative explorations were made into the part played by family life in old age in early sociological surveys, but they were largely concerned with poverty and its effects. By the 1950s, however, there was a growing awareness of the problem presented by increasing numbers of old people. Research carried out at that time by Peter Townsend in Bethnal Green studied the family life of old people.[8] Despite worries that family care might be collapsing, his researches established its central role in the lives of many elderly people. The importance of ease of contact was demonstrated and also the critical part played by the central mother-daughter relationship. Where these family ties were present, provision of basic care, general supervision and nursing in illness was ensured for old people. Whether their role remained intact and their interest in themselves and society was maintained was of course another matter. Old women did better than old men in receiving this type of family support, although men had the advantage of more often having a spouse alive. In Townsend's Bethnal Green group, just under one-fifth of the old people had no surviving children and it is probable that in this country today, up to a quarter of people over 65 have no surviving children. They are without crucial family support and are thus very vulnerable.

Part Played by the Family in Illness

Whenever nursing is required by an old person, whether it is due to illness or the effect of age itself, the family is the first to be asked to give help. The importance of the family in this area was first shown by Townsend and Wedderburn when they were able to demonstrate that the main source of help in sickness was from husbands, wives and children.[9] Housework, cooking and shopping were all undertaken by these helpers. Quite a substantial proportion also relied in times of illness on help from other relatives. There were, however, limits to family care and Townsend found 13 per cent of old people were imposing strain on relatives as a result of incapacity. Amongst married couples, the wife or husband provided care for the sick partner, but this often produced considerable strain on the one who was well. This situation might also apply to siblings living together. A case is remembered of two sisters, one crippled with arthritis and relying entirely on the other for care. Such was the strain on the well sister that eventually she had to be admitted to hospital with heart failure and the crippled sister had to be cared for by the Social Services Department.

Providing basic needs becomes very important during illness. Very often personal bodily care is required and an old person may be very modest in this respect. Some old people refuse to allow anyone except their spouse to wash or bath them, and this is particularly true of men. It is thought improper for another female relative to attend to the bodily functions of an old man. Children may themselves stop short at undertaking such tasks and this produces limitations on what can be done by the family. Old women are in a better position because it is often accepted as natural for a daughter to attend to her needs, but sometimes this means that one member of the family is singled out to carry out more than her fair share of the burden, because an old person will accept no one else. This leads to unequal distribution of responsibility for care and may lead to its breakdown. It is often, therefore, when attending to personal needs that family help falters. This may not always be perceived because domestic tasks may continue to be undertaken very effectively.

The Changing Scene in Family Life

When Townsend did his Bethnal Green survey in the 1950s certain characteristics of family life were described. As mentioned earlier, probably four out of five old people had at least one child; but the general pattern of childbearing then was different to that of today. Marriage was later and child-rearing was spread out over many years. Thus, a man marrying at 25 might not have his last child until he was 39. This applied to women also, although in general, they would be a few years younger. The parents would therefore be in their sixties before the last child reached marrying age and it could be expected that there would be at least one unmarried child at home until both parents were nearing pensionable age. This produced strong ties between a child and parent and with the prolongation into late middle age of parental care of children, it was assumed that the parents would look to and get support from these children when illness arose or infirmity necessitated extra care. There were no doubt exceptions to this pattern, but today the general situation has become quite different. The age of marriage and of childbearing is much lower, although whether this habit persists may depend on contraception. There are now signs, because of its efficiency, that young people are putting off having children early in marriage and are tending to wait until either their own or national economic circumstances are good. Large families are a rarity these days and likely to remain so; most families are complete before the parents have reached the age of 30. Extended childbearing throughout the reproductive years characteristic of earlier generations is now much less common. Efficient contraception also enables those who do not want children to avoid having them altogether, and this will inevitably increase the number of old people without family support.

Townsend commented on the special relationship between unmarried children and their elderly parents. Some of these specifically postponed marriage to look after their parents through a sense of duty. This was particularly strong when one of the parents was dead. For instance, Townsend found that a widow's children delayed marrying, often indefinitely. It appears that this is one of the ways in which a family adapts to the loss of one of its members and compensates the individual who was most affected. Children to some extent substituted for their fathers, but this sense of duty is unlikely to be as strong in present-day society.

Even when the children had left home, there was evidence that they lived in close proximity to their parents. Increased mobility has meant that sons and daughters will now move much greater distances away from their parents. Daughters often have to go to work and this is lessening the opportunity for helping their old parents. Even so, many still do provide care and have merely extended their responsibilities. Old people tend to have a deep attachment to their homes, some of which have housed several generations. This often explains why old people prefer to go on living in these old homes, even when seemingly inconvenient.

It can be argued that these changes may lead to neglect of old people by their families and certainly there are heightened difficulties which will be described in the chapter on social vulnerability. Paradoxically, what is perhaps happening is that families are expecting higher standards for their old people and are demanding an increased level of care. They may be unable to provide this themselves and are looking to statutory care bodies to undertake these responsibilities. There is awareness of the high emotional cost of family care for old people and children may be unwilling to pay this; but associated is the realisation that the standard of care they themselves can provide is not good enough, and not what they would really want for their elderly parents. They look more and more to professional helpers to provide the type of care they think their parents deserve.

Retirement

Life for normal people goes through a series of stages. The early years are spent in education and, hopefully, preparation for a career and the ability to earn a living. There then comes the long period of work and the necessity to provide financially for family and children. Finally, the time arrives as old age is approached when the need to work is no longer present and retirement becomes possible. This is the normal pattern, although there may be many individual variations in timing. The average age for retirement in the UK is 65 years for a man and 60 years for a woman; but these ages are in many ways arbitrary and the tendency is for retirement to take place rather earlier and some men now stop working at 58 or 60 years, often in very good physical and mental health. For economic reasons this trend is likely to continue because of the necessity to provide work for younger members of society, and the persistent problems of unemployment.

Unfortunately, retirement has come to be regarded as synonymous with old age. In many ways it is a pity that the word retirement is used at all in this context, because it implies a withdrawal from activity and reduced participation in the affairs of society. This of course is not so, and should not be the attitude adopted towards the act of giving up paid work. It is becoming increasingly recognised that there is a 'young' old age, usually between 65 and 75 years and an 'old' old age from 75 years onwards. For many people the period of 'young' old age can be the best and happiest time of life. Some will wish to continue working, albeit at a slower and more relaxed rate, whereas others may be glad to give up the responsibility of a job and concentrate on other interests, hobbies and pleasures. Many a man has considered retirement to be the most fulfilled part of his life and has wondered how he ever had the time to hold down a full-time job. Retirement then should be a very positive event and should be looked upon as a new adventure. It can be a time of life when, free from the constraints of earning a living, a person can spend time on activities which had previously been impossible. Whether the period after 65 years is one of continuing work or positive retirement, successful and happy living during this period depends on certain basic requirements and some essential adjustments. A person must have health, sufficient interests, and if possible, a freedom from financial worry. Emotional, environmental and physical adjustments need to be made. The foundation for all this can be laid down before the actual event of retirement and entry into old age should really be a continuation of a successful life pattern. People do not change when they arrive at their 65th birthday, but fundamentally continue to enjoy and be interested in life.

Hopefully, a person arrives at retirement healthy, and in this sense early retirement may be advantageous. Most doctors will have seen patients with some degree of incapacity struggling on to reach their 65th birthday, only to live for a relatively short time thereafter; whereas, if retirement had been arranged earlier, perhaps a longer and happier period would have been achieved. Good health, however, needs maintaining. Old people need to be aware of the hazards of disease, particularly the cumulative effect of minor illness. Problems need reporting in sufficient time to allow effective action to be taken. Special care should be taken of ears, eyes, feet and teeth; obesity should be avoided and the dangers of smoking and over-eating appreciated.

There are the problems of hypothermia, falls and faulty nutrition. The need for adequate sleep is important, but old people often need far less than is supposed. Mental and physical exercise is necessary to avoid boredom but psychological adjustment must be made to the physical restrictions which are inevitable as age advances. Some old people worry about the problem of sex and it is now well established that sexual activity can go on well into old age and a retained interest in sexuality is in no way abnormal. People vary in their needs, of course, and the marital pair must recognise the possible difference in each other's requirements.

As mentioned earlier, the financial resources of old people are often very limited. This may improve as superannuation schemes become more widespread and the benefits of earnings-related pensions work through. Financial worry is, however, very real and might be helped if old people availed themselves more fully of additional benefits.

The interests of old people usually reflect those of earlier years and these should be maintained. It is not uncommon, however, for an elderly person to take up quite new activities. These are wide-ranging and reflect the general variety of human interest. Some learn new languages and even take degrees. The less ambitious are content to spend more time gardening or continue with their interest in, for instance, music. The possibilities are endless, but perhaps it is very important to belong to some sort of community organisation. This may be a society of some kind, or a church or voluntary organisation. The stimulus of meeting people and creating friendships is very valuable.

The type of environment in which an old person lives is also important to his health and happiness. It is obviously quite wrong for a man with a tendency to bronchitis to move on retirement to a country cottage 600 feet above sea level where the winter is cold and there is the risk of isolation. It is a good idea to think about the type of house in which a person is going to live after retirement well before the event. It should be easily run and adequately and cheaply heated. A bungalow is often ideal but is not always popular with elderly people as 'stair legs', so necessary for visiting others and getting about generally, are lost and many people feel vulnerable sleeping on the ground floor. The garden obviously should not be too large and keeping it tidy should be as easy as possible. Access to public transport, shops, entertainment and medical services must also be considered.

Apart from these environmental considerations, certain mental and emotional adjustments need to be made towards retirement. To cease being a productive member of society can sometimes be traumatic. The status and protection offered by holding a job is lost and a person has to learn to stand on his own feet as an individual. He may, however, lose his self-respect and feel he has no purpose in life. An insight into these problems is very necessary if mental health is to be preserved. Emotional conflicts sometimes arise within a marriage at this time and this can be understood when a man who has been used to being at work each day suddenly finds himself around the house and continually in contact with (or under the feet of) his wife. This may lead to accentuation of existing conflicts. The wife may find that she now has to attend to extra domestic chores, such as making additional meals, whilst the husband does nothing but pursue his own interests. She may feel that she is not benefiting from retirement and considerable mutual adjustment and communication may be necessary to avoid building up resentments. A man, on the other hand, may find it hard to adjust to his new role of domestic partner rather than breadwinner and he may need tactful support from his wife to retain his self-confidence.

Education about these problems is often helpful and there has developed in recent years the idea that there should be some sort of formal preparation for retirement. Pre-retirement classes are now run by Education Authorities, often in partnership with industry. The timing of these courses is variable but perhaps they should start about five years before retirement with another shorter course a few weeks before the actual time. Evidence has been produced for the usefulness of this type of exercise and it should certainly help to encourage positive thinking towards successful retirement.

Change in Society

This century has seen many social changes. One feature which has affected old people is the development of a youth-orientated society. The entertainment and fashion world is totally focused on the young and the elderly may often feel left out. Despite this, the young themselves, with their healthy interest in community action, are sympathetic to the old and do much in voluntary work to assist.

There has grown a more materialistic outlook towards life, with little emphasis on the old-fashioned moral and spiritual standards still very much alive in the minds of old people. Television and the mass media have been very active and powerful propagandists in this sense.

Transport has become considerably easier and it is now possible for people to travel with ease to many parts of the world. Millions spend holidays on the sunshine beaches of the Mediterranean and occasionally the elderly can benefit from these amenities. On the other hand, increased mobility has meant that large dormitory housing estates have mushroomed on the outer fringes of towns and cities, denuding the centres of population, and leaving them to the old and the poor.

The working week has been reduced and most people now work shorter hours with more time for relaxation and enjoyment. Despite this, unemployment has become a permanent feature of modern society and to relieve this, early retirement has been encouraged. This has brought with it an increase in the psychological trauma of fit people suddenly finding themselves redundant and facing a lower standard of living, although hopefully this may not be the norm.

The creation of the Welfare State and the enormous advances in medical care and of social security have greatly helped old people, and many more now live to extreme old age. This has caused increased economic strains on society. The status of women has also changed. There has been a justifiable fight for equal rights and equal opportunities. This may have brought with it the necessity for them to accept responsibilities which previously they did not possess and many women are now wage-earners on whom the family depends economically. Women are no longer as freely available to attend to family needs and particularly to provide care for elderly relatives. The technological revolution has provided many labour-saving devices, but these are expensive in both fuel and capital outlay. The poor in the community, who often include the elderly, are unable to avail themselves of these developments. Environmentally, towns and cities are increasingly being replanned and this has brought with it vast developments and changes in urban living. Until recently, the sociological implications of these happenings have been largely overlooked. The poor, including many elderly people, have probably suffered more than any other group. The massive and necessary slum clearance programmes of the last quarter of a century have caused large movements of population. People have been moved from homes where they have lived for many years and have been placed in other quite different areas. To the old it has often been traumatic, particularly if the move was, for instance, to high-rise flats. Fortunately, these problems are being recognised by planners and politicians who now accept the enormous responsibility they carry for the quality of people's lives when they redesign the fabric of our cities and towns.

There are also the modern features of emigration and immigration. Many healthy young adults have emigrated abroad, leaving their elderly behind. Sadness and loneliness are often the lot of these old people. At the same time there has been the arrival of immigrants from Commonwealth countries. There is now in this country a multiracial society with all the inherent challenges of integration and education. The new arrivals move into the poorer inner city or town areas and often into old terraced houses. These are frequently the type also occupied by the indigenous elderly who are usually less adaptable and may find integration difficult.

With all these changes, the elderly may well tend to be forgotten. Fortunately, groups exist which strive for their rights and ensure that they have a voice in how affairs are managed. But what role does society expect old people to perform? Perhaps there has always been an ambivalent attitude as to what this should be. Ideally, work should be available for those who want it and are capable; integration into the community and social life should be the aim. This is the goal which many ageing people strive to attain, but obstacles are increasingly being constructed by society. Nothing is expected of old people economically and they no longer contribute to the work-force because it is the young who have priority in this respect. It is left to the old to be the backbone of voluntary societies, churches and social clubs. Their experience and judgement is valued still in these fields and they are able to contribute socially in these ways. Many chairmen and secretaries of amateur organisations and football clubs are elderly men who have done the job for years. They themselves enjoy the activities and feel fulfilled in undertaking them, but perhaps this role too is disappearing. There are many more elderly people around and not all can be secretaries of local organisations. Are they now unwanted in the community? Society must ask itself this question. Hopefully, the answer will be no, and opportunities will be created for them to contribute and be involved, instead of withdrawing into the background and waiting for the professional services to take over. The young elderly may be very important in this respect as they usually retain the health and energy necessary to organise community self-support activities.

Notes

1. P. Townsend and D. Wedderburn, *The Aged in the Welfare State* (London, Bell, 1965).
2. Audrey Hunt, *The Elderly at Home* (Office of Population Censuses and Surveys, Social Survey Division) (London, HMSO,1978).
3. A.C. Bebbington, 'The Elderly at Home Survey. Changes in the Provision of Domiciliary Social Services to the Elderly over Fourteen Years', unpublished discussion paper 87, DHSS.
4. Unpublished DHSS Discussion Document, 'Conference on the Elderly', 26 July 1977.
5. Rosamund Gruer, *Needs of the Elderly in the Scottish Borders* (Edinburgh, Scottish Home and Health Department, 1975).
6. E.I. Williams *et al.*, 'Sociomedical Study of Patients over 75 in General Practice', *British Medical Journal*, vol.2 (1972), pp.445-8.
7. Hunt, *The Elderly at Home.*
8. P. Townsend, *The Family Life of Old People* (London, Routledge and Kegan Paul, 1957; also Pelican Books).
9. Townsend and Wedderburn, *The Aged in the Welfare State.*

Further Reading

Eric Butterworth and David Weir (eds.), *The Sociology of Modern Britain* (London, Fontana/Collins, 1972).

Preparation for Retirement: New Approaches (Beth Johnson Foundation Publications, 1976).

PART TWO: CONTEMPORARY PROBLEMS

The features of old age so far described can be said to be those normally found in present-day society. A situation exists where larger numbers of people are achieving the age of 65 and beyond. With this increase in numbers there has also grown a better understanding of the nature of ageing in the community, but the pattern of care available is still very much at the point to which it had evolved by the mid-twentieth century. This is often inadequate in present-day circumstances. Family responsibility is still considered paramount in the provision of care for old people, but families are probably finding this more difficult. The situation presented by these facts, namely difficulties in the provision of care and the increased possibility of social breakdown, will now be considered.

5 PROVISION OF SERVICES

There is a story which is often told and which has now become classic. It concerns a doctor who was called to see an old man late on a Friday afternoon. It was winter and the doctor was tired after a particularly arduous week. He arrived at the house to find an old man in his seventies who had been unwell for some weeks. He now had bronchitis which had followed an earlier cold. He lived alone in a run-down terraced house with little in the way of amenities. The doctor was greeted somewhat aggressively by relatives of the old man who had just called to see him: they were very disturbed by the situation and felt unable to give adequate care. Despite the fact that nobody had bothered to do anything earlier about their ageing grandfather's plight, they now demanded that 'something should be done' and preferably that hospital admission should be arranged immediately.

Dismayed at finding a circumstance of which he previously knew nothing, the doctor wearily realised that he was faced with the complex task of arranging for the care of his old patient. It was obvious that someone needed to look after him, but that the poor social state made this difficult at home. The relatives were plainly reluctant to help and the doctor, after assessing the patient and giving him emergency treatment, started the frustrating round of telephone calls. The hospital geriatric ward was full to overflowing as a result of the inclement winter condition. More admissions could be expected over the weekend often with more severe medical problems than the old man with his bronchitis. 'Could the doctor hold out for a day or two' was their plea. The Social Services Department had by this time closed, and an hour passed before the social worker on duty could be found. 'This is a medical, not a social problem', she insisted and added that it was too late to arrange for help in the house and the welfare homes were also full. Frustration was mounting. The doctor asked the relatives if they would take charge until the morning but in this particular case they could not offer any assistance and the doctor was left with the prospect of arranging emergency admission. The hospital of course ultimately took the patient, but a bed was used which might have been better utilised by another person.

Anyone working in the community knows the type of situation described and the story contains no exaggerations. The services available in different areas do, of course, vary. Sometimes it is possible to provide emergency social care and often relatives manage despite severe difficulties. But they frequently feel that they are not providing a good enough standard of care and realise that the situation can only deteriorate. Hospitals in the end will admit this type of patient, but how much better it would have been if the situation could have been prevented or foreseen, and treatment and care instituted at an earlier stage.

The Triangle of Care

One of the principles which the above story illustrates about caring for old people in the community is the close link which exists between medical and social problems. Both are often present at the same time and it is usually merely a matter of degree as to whether the patient needs primarily medical (and this includes nursing) care or primarily social services (i.e. provision of basic care). When a person needs care in the overall sense, there are three places where this can be given. These are in his own home, in welfare accommodation or in the hospital. The place in which it is most appropriate for him to be really depends on the balance between the medical and social needs and also the possibilities of whether either or both of these can be effectively provided for in his own home. Care in a patient's home or in a welfare home is referred to as community care, the social aspects being the responsibility of the Local Authority Social Services and the medical aspects those of the primary health care team. For convenience, warden-supervised sheltered housing is regarded in this chapter as synonymous with the patient's own home. It is of fundamental importance that these three places of care should be used appropriately. As Figure 5.1 shows, they form a triangle and should be interrelated with a free flow of patients from one to the other. Thus, a patient may be admitted to hospital for acute care but may return to the community and his home via the half-way stage of a welfare home when social problems need resolving. Alternatively, he may need only short-stay welfare home accommodation to overcome an acute social problem. Several combinations and possibilities therefore exist. This chapter is primarily concerned with the actual problems which currently exist in the provision of services to the elderly. The details of the community services themselves will be described fully later in the sections on contemporary solutions and resources available. In practice, difficulties occur in all three places of care and in what might be called the fourth side of the triangle which is co-operation between the workers in each.

Figure 5.1: Triangle of Care

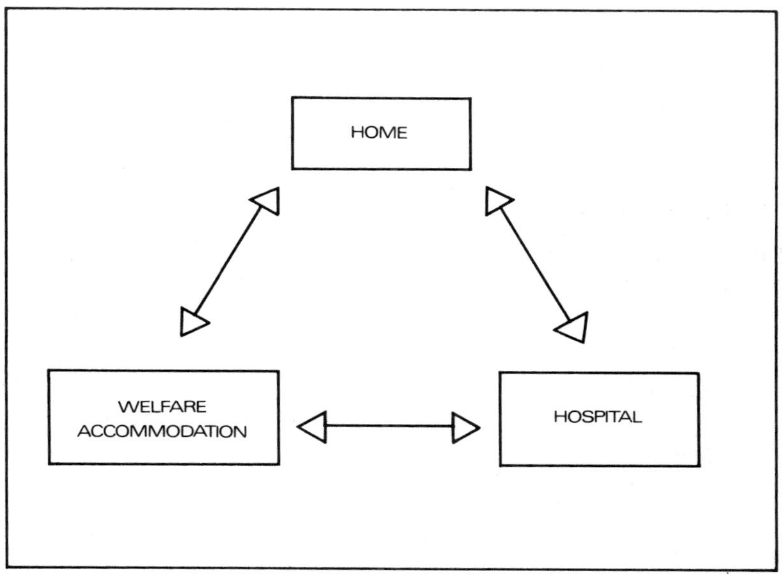

These will now be discussed in more detail.

Care in the Home

The difficulties of the services caring for old people in the community are extensive and can have several causes. Some are due to the attitudes and experience of those working with old people. There may be doctors who have little interest in the elderly and lack training in geriatric care. They may therefore have a poor appreciation of the natural history of ageing and the sometimes atypical characteristics of disease in this age group. Mental illness in old age is a good example of a subject which, although requiring considerable skill to manage, especially in its acute crisis form, has attracted little attention. Often such important things as resettlement of patients discharged from hospital and their continuing care and rehabilitation are ignored. Such attitudes are reinforced if there is insufficient domiciliary nursing help or a non-existent rehabilitation service in the community. The standard of medical and social care available for old people in the community has been criticised for some time. Indeed, as far back as the spring of 1972 the Royal College of General Practitioners received a copy of the critical publication *Age Concern on Health.*[1] This prompted the College to set up a small working party to examine published reports on geriatric care in the community and to suggest ways in which it could be improved. The resulting paper, 'Geriatric Care in General Practice' by A.E. Elliott and J.S.K. Stevenson, began by summarising the criticisms specifically levelled at general practice by the Age Concern report and these were as follows:[2]

1. The organisation of general practice has made it more difficult for elderly patients to consult their doctors, for example by the centralisation of consulting premises and the growth of appointments systems.
2. The general practitioner's changing attitude towards home visiting makes the geriatric patient reluctant to call the doctor, and the general practitioner less likely to call on the patient.
3. Transport difficulties make access to the general practitioner and the pharmacist more difficult, especially for the very old and those living alone.
4. There appears to be an increasing use of repeat prescriptions in place of consultations.
5. There is disquiet about the increasing chance of seeing different doctors within a group practice.
6. There is often lack of continuity of care when elderly patients are discharged from hospital or from convalescence.
7. Some complain of the lack of continuing supervision by general practitioners and health visitors of the very old and high risk groups.
8. General worries exist among the elderly as to how they should act in emergencies.

Elliott and Stevenson went on to make suggestions about recognising old people in need and ways of improving practice organisation. Unfortunately, only patchy progress has been made in implementing their excellent proposals.

Other difficulties arise because it is sometimes not possible to create suitable environmental arrangements for old people. Rehousing or adaptation of existing houses may be difficult. Transport may be hard to organise. Communications such as telephone installation may be regarded as too expensive. Basic social services such as home helps and 'meals on wheels' may be inadequate and care on a longer-term basis may be unavailable in some areas.

There may be too few trained workers available to deal with the complex variety of incidents presented by old people and there are also financial considerations affecting the standard of care. How much help should be given and how much money should be spent? These are difficult questions to answer but obviously a balance is necessary. L.J. Opit, writing in 1977, reports an investigation into the cost of domiciliary care of 139 elderly sick patients by the Home Nursing Service.[3] The data suggest that there may be little economic advantage in home care for elderly seriously disabled people. The revenue costs of domiciliary care were equal to or even greater than the average hospital care of such patients. It must be remembered that Opit took the highest domiciliary care costs and the lowest hospital care costs. Whether these findings will be confirmed remains to be seen, and in any case there are other considerations to be taken note of when deciding where it is best to nurse a very sick old person, such as his own wishes and the expected duration of his illness or disability. Nevertheless, financial considerations will continue to influence the quality of domiciliary care given to old people.

Welfare Home and Sheltered Care

Welfare homes can be general, catering for all types of old people, or specifically designed for certain groups such as the mentally handicapped. In some areas the number of places available is insufficient for the demand and sometimes they are not used appropriately. A common fault is lack of flow between welfare home and hospital and vice versa. Many homes are increasingly being used for old people who need a high degree of nursing care. For this reason some argue that it would be better if welfare accommodation was administered by Area Health Authorities and became integrated into the health care services.

Warden-supervised housing units also pose difficulties. The residents of these are often very old and a high proportion are in their eighties. This produces extra burdens and strains on the warden, particularly when as many as 100 old people may have access to her services through an intercom system. Perhaps some young elderly people should be introduced into sheltered housing schemes to help with warden duties. This could well provide a worthwhile task for a fit person of 65 to 70.

Hospital Services

Hospital departments of geriatric medicine have three perennial problems: maintaining adequate staffing levels, existing in substandard accommodation, and having enough beds available to meet the high demand. It is undoubtedly difficult to attract doctors and nurses to work with elderly patients. There are many reasons for this but one is the poor state and isolated position of many geriatric wards. Considering the actual fabric of some departments of geriatric medicine, it is surprising to note how much excellent work is being undertaken. In May 1971 the South East Metropolitan Hospital Board published a report on its geriatric services.[4] The deficiencies exposed showed the poor state of the actual hospitals themselves and this was highlighted by the fact that several of these had seen previous service as infectious disease or chest hospitals and 18 had originated as workhouses or public assistance institutions. Fifteen of the latter were over 100 years old, the oldest being 177 years, and even this was not the most elderly geriatric hospital in this country.

The so-called 'blocked bed', a possibly unfortunate term used to describe the situation of some old person using (and presumably needing) the bed over a long period, really describes the situation of beds filled with patients who could more appropriately be cared for either at home or in a welfare home. Skilled medical and nursing care may not be necessary and the reason for hospital residence is basically social. This affects community care because it blocks the free flow of patients round the triangle of care. It is, however, not only a feature of departments of geriatric medicine. Murphy did a cross-section survey of 325 surgical and orthopaedic beds and 43 of the 265 occupied beds were filled by patients who had no medical need to be in an acute ward.[5] The patients had been in hospital for a median time of 40 weeks up to the survey dates. Of the 43 patients, 11 were awaiting transfer to a geriatric ward, 13 to community residential care and 7 to their own homes. There was no plan for discharge or transfer of the remaining twelve. There was a high risk of becoming a long-stay patient for social reasons in the case of women over 75 years of age who were living alone and had been admitted to hospital with a fractured femur or other trauma. Murphy considered that action necessary to help the situation should include:

(a) changing attitudes to the solving of social case problems;
(b) revising procedures of assessment and planning of future care;
(c) improving team work and record-keeping within the hospital and community services;
(d) providing a better balance of acute, medium- and long-stay

hospital beds;

(e) putting more resources into rehabilitation.

Medical wards also have similar predicaments. Christine McArdle *et al.*, during a nine-month study found that 160 out of 482 bed weeks in an acute medical ward were accounted for by 11 patients who no longer needed to be there.[6] She comments that this was unsatisfactory both for the 11 patients concerned and for those patients requiring admission for whom beds were blocked. This situation can sometimes lead to demarcation disputes between consultants, particularly in such grey areas as psychogeriatrics, where perhaps neither geriatricians nor psychiatrists want to accept responsibility or have adequate resources. Skilled medical and nursing care can certainly extend an old person's life considerably and great care is necessary before deciding that a long-stay bed is the best answer to a particular circumstance.

It is not the general intention of this book to describe in detail the services provided for old people by the hospital as they have been described excellently elsewhere and the main emphasis is here given to care in the community. Nevertheless, a very close link between these two areas exists and there is a very necessary partnership between the two. Everyone working in the community must be aware of the facilities provided by the hospital and these will therefore be briefly described at this point.

Despite the inherent difficulties, the hospital departments of geriatric medicine are expanding and developing their services. They provide specialist care for old people; although it must be remembered that many in the elderly age group are also looked after by other doctors such as psychiatrists or surgeons in other parts of the hospital. The specialist department of geriatric medicine is organised and supervised by one or more consultant physicians in geriatric medicine. Patients may be referred by a general practitioner to the out-patients' department or can be seen at home by the specialist on a domiciliary consultation. Direct admission is usually available for patients over a certain age (usually 72 or 73 years old) in an emergency. Once admitted, the patient arrives at an acute geriatric ward, usually situated in a general hospital. The principle of programmed patient care is the feature of modern geriatric medicine. In the initial stage, the patient's medical and social problems are analysed and treatment started. He may then be able to return home or may need further rehabilitaton and may need to be moved to the geriatric rehabilitation ward. This may involve a stay of two or three months, but usually the patient can then return either to his own home, or be admitted to a welfare home. Considerable medical and social effort often goes into preparing the patient for discharge after rehabilitation. Sometimes, however, patients remain sufficiently disabled to make it impossible to discharge them back into the community. Here long-term hospital care becomes necessary. Continuing care in hospital is an important part of the service provided by departments of geriatric medicine and one where help from volunteers is encouraged. The wards should be as 'non-hospital' as possible, with opportunities for recreation and privacy.

In addition to acute long-term and rehabilitation admission, most geriatric departments will admit patients for holiday relief to help relatives. Just how appropriate it is to bring patients into hospital purely for 'holidays' is debatable. Purposive admission for the benefit of the patient is of course the ideal. Relief for the relatives will then hopefully result from the patient's improvement. Intermittent admission can also be arranged for patients who need to be helped over some domestic or social hardship.

Most geriatric services now provide day hospital facilities. The prime purpose of these is to continue with rehabilitation and maintain progress previously made in hospital. It also provides these services for those who have not been in-patients. Relief is provided for relatives in this way as patients are taken to the hospital in the morning and brought back in the late afternoon by ambulance. Medical and nursing services are available without the necessity for direct admission. Early discharge from hospital is often facilitated and resettlement made easier by the day hospital. Finally, the geriatric services are very important in training. Instruction in geriatric care is provided for medical students, doctors, nurses, social workers and ancillary staff.

Co-ordination

The professional care of the elderly is basically the responsibility of the medical services who are concerned with health, and the social services who are concerned with social well-being. Administratively, these two partners are quite separate. Since the recent reorganisation of the National Health Service, both the hospital and general practitioner services have become the responsibility of the Area Health Authorities and are ultimately administered by the Department of Health and Social Security. The Social Services Departments are administered by Local Authorities. The merging of the hospital and GP service under the Area Health Authority should at least have made co-operation between them more effective. The new Family Practitioner Committees responsible for general practitioners remain, however, autonomous bodies and new arrangements have made little impact on the work and administration of general practice. Developments in general practice and particularly advances in the provision of care and extended teamwork will have to come from doctors themselves. Research, perhaps in university departments of general practice, should point the way. By example and teaching, these departments may hopefully influence the practice and facilities provided by their colleagues.

Co-operation between health workers and social workers seems even more difficult to achieve. Admittedly, the Social Service Departments have responsibilities apart from the elderly, but occasionally there is the impression that social workers are not interested in co-operation with health workers when dealing with old people. No doubt there are regional variations in this. Many authorities have been so burdened by financial restriction that only very limited services can be offered and therefore they are not searching for any possible extension of their activities. Nevertheless, co-operation will eventually have to be achieved as the whole area of community care for old people must be a combined medical and social exercise. Such projects as that undertaken by the Caversham Group Practice team and the National Institute of Social Work Training have given a lead in clarifying the nature of the partnership between social workers and doctors.[7]

Built into the reorganised National Health Service administrative structure are opportunities for representatives of hospital and general practice to contribute to various levels of planning. Planning care teams for the elderly have been established and have serving on them geriatricians, general practitioners, hospital and community nurses, health visitors, dentists, representatives of Social Services and Housing Departments and administrators. These meet to plan and co-ordinate the services to the elderly in the area. Although undoubtedly successful overall, certain weaknesses are becoming apparent in these planning teams. One of these is that they have perhaps inevitably come to be dominated by the problems of the hospital. General practitioner members also have some difficulty in the sense that they are there primarily as representatives and are not able to commit any of their colleagues to various aspects of community care. They therefore have very little opportunity to influence directly what goes on, apart from in their own practices. Development will need to take place by more discussion between family doctors about services to the elderly, ideally at post-graduate centres. Discussion at planning team meetings is helpful, but co-operation really needs to start at ground level if fully comprehensive community care is to be achieved. Hopeful signs of improved co-operation between social services and medical services exist in the government schemes for joint financing projects. Area Health Authorities and Social Services have joint consultative arrangements, but it will probably take some time before the impact of these developments is realised at the level of patient care.

Expectations

Colouring all these difficulties are the changes which have been occurring in society, particularly in attitudes of families towards their elderly relatives. There is an increased expectation of the standards of professional care which should be available to old people. This adds to the burdens of community workers when these hopes, and sometimes demands, cannot be satisfied. Friction undoubtedly occurs when, for instance, hospital admission is unavailable or domiciliary services are inadequate.

Notes

1. *Age Concern on Health* (London National Old People's Welfare Council, 1972).
2. A.E. Elliott and J.S.K. Stevenson, 'Geriatric Care in General Practice', *Journal of the Royal College of General Practitioners*, vol.23 (1973), pp.615-25.
3. L.J. Opit, 'Domiciliary Care for the Elderly Sick. Economical Neglect?', *British Medical Journal*, vol.1 (1977), pp.30-3.
4. Department of Services for the Elderly and Elderly Confused in South East Metropolitan Hospital Region, 1970.
5. F.W. Murphy, 'Blocked Beds', *British Medical Journal*, vol.4 (1975), pp.568-9.
6. Christine McArdle, J.C. Wiley and W.D. Alexander, 'Geriatric Patients in an Acute Medical Ward', *British Medical Journal*, vol.4 (1975), pp.568-9.
7. E. Matilda Goldeberg and Jane E. Neill, *Social Work in General Practice* (London, George Allen and Unwin, 1972).

Further Reading

J.C. Brocklehurst, 'Ageing and Health' in David Hobman (ed.), *The Social Challenge of Ageing* (London, Croom Helm, 1978), ch.5.

M. Keith Thompson, *Geriatrics and the General Practitioner Team* (Baltimore, Williams and Wilkins, 1969).

6 SOCIAL VULNERABILITY

In Chapter 4 an account was given of the situation of old people in society and it will be perceived that social problems in old age are, if not inevitable, always a possibility. In social terms the word 'problem' is of course not easily defined because how a situation is viewed depends very much on the position of the observer. An objective outsider may see 'a problem' which is seemingly non-existent in the eyes of the person actually living in the situation. Thus, an old person with an apparent social problem may in fact be content with his way of life and may resent interference. Even so, real difficulties do occur and are often linked with illness and both doctor and social worker are subsequently involved in joint management.

Social Independence

Most old people are socially independent and live happily in the community. The basic requirements described earlier are satisfied and amenities are present to enable a full and satisfying standard of life to be enjoyed. If not provided by the old people themselves, the basic necessities are given by relatives, neighbours and friends. An old person then is usually happy in this state of equilibrium although perhaps it is occasionally only maintained with some difficulty.

What Goes Wrong?

Two types of situation can arise which cause a change in the social equilibrium of an old person. Both produce domestic deterioration – one insidiously and the other dramatically. The first is where, although basic care is still being given, a time arrives when certain tasks, necessary activities and even hobbies are becoming too demanding for the old person himself to undertake and there is then a slow but steady lowering of the quality of living, although this may not yet be appreciated. The second is when a crisis arises because there is sudden breakdown in the provision of basic care.

Isaacs and Neville, in their study of the Scottish health services, detail in their book *The Measurement of Need in Old People* three categories of old person.[1] The first is the *protected* where the old person is in an institution and therefore protected from social problems. The second is the *defended* where the old person is cared for by relatives and thus in a state of social equilibrium and defended from social problems. The third is the *defeated*, and this is where the old person fails to receive basic care or where relatives are suffering an intolerable strain in providing it.

The concepts of the defended and the defeated are important because with a defensible situation, help can be given to maintain the old person in the community, usually by providing short interval or critical interval care; the defeated position usually requires admission to a protected environment either in the hospital or welfare home. Isaacs and Neville found that for every severely disabled old person in hospital, there were two at home with a similar degree of disability and therefore often on the brink of changing from being defended to being defeated. This means that care is still being given but presumably at great cost to the provider.

It is with the defeated situation that the doctor or social worker is usually involved; but the process of change from a defended equilibrium to the defeated or near-defeated position is often gradual and constitutes the first of the types of social breakdown which may require help. The actual defeat is usually a crisis and this is the second type of situation needing help. These two will be discussed separately although they may be part of the same process. The first, which involves non-crisis problems, may only be the forerunner of the second. Recognition of problems in the non-crisis group at an early enough stage can, however, sometimes prevent breakdown.

Non-crisis Difficulties

In Tables 4.1 and 4.2 (pp. 45-6) some examples of personal and domestic tasks essential to normal living were listed. Although inability to undertake any of these can produce hardships, failure to be able to perform basic functions, such as washing and feeding, are the most serious. It is possible that where there is difficulty with one task, there is likely to be similar difficulty with another. Indeed, certain tasks can be grouped so that when one of the tasks cannot be performed, it is likely that the others cannot be performed either. For instance in personal tasks, those related to mobility in the home, for example climbing stairs, getting around the house, getting in and out of bed and going to the lavatory, form a natural group. Similarly, there is a second group involved with mobility outside the house and with those tasks involving the whole body, for instance bathing, cutting toe-nails and using public transport. Finally, a group can be formed out of tasks involving physical manipulation of the hands, for instance shaving, washing and feeding.

It is likely that a person who experiences difficulty with one task, also experiences difficulty with others in a group. The recognition of these associations may be important to the social worker when assessing functional ability. These observations were originally made by Barlow and Matthews[2] in their study of Audrey Hunt's report, *The Elderly at Home.*[3]

Grouping can also be made for domestic tasks, although this is complicated by sex roles. For example, it is traditional for women to be associated with cooking and washing, and men to be associated with doing minor repairs. Even so, broad divisions can be made between ligher and heavier housework. It is often important to recognise that if an old person is finding difficulty in one task he may also be finding difficulty with other tasks. The full extent of the problem may be unperceived unless this is recognised.

Many of these problems may be minor at first, and there are numerous examples. It might become impossible to continue taking the dog for a walk; or the garden becomes too difficult to manage and hence lawn-mowing and weeding are neglected. Slowly household maintenance may also suffer and eventually care of shoes and clothes may be overlooked. Long-distance mobility may become impossible. A visit may be made to the local shops but longer journeys to buy special items may be avoided; hobbies and visits to clubs may be discontinued. Help for this type of problem is usually provided by neighbours and relatives, but if no one is available, standards begin to fall.

Some problems are more subtle and hence more difficult for a family to solve. It may not be easy to perceive that old people are failing to keep up with changing economic circumstances, and are not easily assimilating new information. Thus, pension rates change, licensing fees for television are raised and these facts need to be understood by an old person. Poverty has long been a problem of old age and this may not only be due to a lack of money but also, for example, to having an expenditure ridiculously out of proportion to the necessities. The house may be too large and a burden to maintain. Some old people have financial commitments to relatives which are obviously unfair and cause a considerable amount of stress and worry. On the other hand, many of these old people come from a thrifty generation who have always been taught to save for a rainy day and now, in extreme old age when this is obviously non-existent, they still feel the necessity to save or at least not spend extravagantly. They are reluctant to buy food, clothes and fuel for heat even though they have quite adequate resources to do this.

Savings preclude help from the state and it is sometimes hard for relatives to persuade an old person to spend some of the reserve money on the basic necessities of life.

Retirement itself may bring problems. A man's adjustment to being constantly around the house and his wife's acceptance of it is not easily achieved. Quarrels may ensue and result in rifts within a family with long-lasting repercussions on the standard of care being given. Family disputes can take other forms and it is well known that as age advances, some old people can become extremely unreasonable. Difficult character traits which were perhaps accepted in earlier years can become exaggerated to such an extent that an old person can become awkward and vindictive. Particular likes or dislikes can be taken to certain relatives and neighbours and sometimes the elderly may be in a position to make life extremely difficult for these people. The net result is a lack of sympathy and the old person fails to receive necessary help.

Minor mental deterioration may not be recognised and subtle behavioural change may pass unnoticed until it becomes a serious problem. A good example of this is a tendency to hoard. In the early stages this may amount to nothing more than an exaggeration of a natural instinct to gather in supplies of food, or an old man's eccentric hobby of collecting newspapers or periodicals. But once the house becomes a fantastic jungle of irrelevant items, things have gone too far and the situation is abnormal.

Sexual problems sometimes arise and an old man may become more demanding on his now unsympathetic wife. His attentions are perhaps turned on other women in the immediate circle and although this is often regarded as playfulness and treated as a joke, it can be extremely embarrassing. The family tends to cover up the real nature of the problem in these circumstances and help is hard to give.

The phenomenon of the captive spouse is also not infrequently seen. As time goes on, one member of the marital pair may become ill and need looking after. This involves the other partner in a considerable additional burden. Not only are there the normal household duties but also the extra commitments of caring physically and environmentally for the sick partner. This creates the situation where the well member has to withdraw from all previous outside activities and care becomes a full-time occupation. There are times in late old age when a man or woman may be working harder than at any other time in earlier life and although the situation may appear to be very well managed, it must be realised that this is happening at great cost. Social as well as physical help is often desperately needed. Particularly tragic is the plight of aged parents with a physically or mentally handicapped son or daughter living with them. The offspring is often ageing as well and needing more, and not less, help.

Outside influences can also affect the standard of life of old people. National strikes, for instance, of power workers and ambulance drivers can have a much more damaging effect on the aged than on other sections of the community. In Britain today, there is a multiracial society. At present the proportion of old people is not high amongst immigrants but this will change and may bring special problems.

These are examples of social problems which are often part of a gradual decline. The process is slow. It might take years before it is realised how far the standard of life has fallen. As with illness, many problems are unreported and are often multiple. Some are quite intractable and these may be accepted as such and not cause difficulty. Trigger difficulties of relatively minor degree can, however, sometimes plunge the situation into crisis and it is necessary to watch out for these. It is surprising how, for instance, equilibrium exists despite obvious overcrowding in a household, the real problem only being perceived when it is realised that it is responsible for a child's persistent truancy from school. Because of the presence of aged grandparents at home the child can find no privacy and seeks it in the solitude of a friend's house in the daytime.

Acute Social Crises

Acute crises occur socially when there is a breakdown in the provision of basic care and action is then usually necessary by the caring services. The nature of the crisis usually depends on the underlying causes. These can broadly be divided into problems with the old person, problems with the helpers, problems with the environment and failures in communication. There is considerable overlap between these factors but for convenience they will be examined separately.

Patient or Client Problems

Old people may be living alone or with relatives. Where there is help in the house, difficulties occur when the level of basic care required is such that it is impossible for the helpers to cope. When an old person lives alone it is the fact that he can no longer self-care which produces the trouble. In both situations where the problem is patient- or client-centred, it is usually illness which precipitates the breakdown. This can be physical or mental and may be major or minor, and it often does not matter which; the important thing being that as a result basic care can no longer be provided. Minor episodes of influenza or gastro-enteritis can have the same effect as heart failure. Usually major illness such as stroke demands immediate admission to hospital, and this temporarily eases the situation, but hardship can arise when this type of patient is discharged home. However, sometimes even minor illness can result in the patient being admitted to hospital as basic social care is not possible at home. Progressive illnesses such as chronic nerve degeneration involve slow deterioration and crisis then occurs less obviously, but even so a point is reached where care is needed. Terminal illness may also produce similar urgent problems. Falls and accidents may bring sudden social incapacity. An old lady might be managing very well until a slip on the ice results in a fractured wrist. Treatment at a local casualty department is easy but the patient is quite unable to cope when she arrives back home. Sometimes admission to a welfare home is required, though often only for a short time. Other injuries, such as a fractured femur, demand a longer period of rehabilitation. Mental illness frequently causes social problems, and these are discussed in Chapter 13. It is not uncommon for old people to attempt suicide and this may be a symptom of their inability to cope with the demands of basic living. Behavioural problems may also present as acute social crises. Failing vision and deafness may render the patient incapable of self-care, especially when handling of drugs and self-administering of treatment are needed. All the situations discussed in the section on non-crisis situations may flare up into acute crisis. Particularly vulnerable are patients who are bedfast and housefast.

Helper Problems

Patient difficulties can have an effect on helpers and on some more than others. Admission to hospital geriatric departments is often due to friends and relatives being unable to cope at home. Sanford found this to be so in 12 per cent of all geriatric admissions to University College Hospital, London, and to the Whittington Hospital.[4] The person principally involved with home support was interviewed in 50 such cases. The causes of inability to cope were identified on a qualitative and quantitative basis. The supporters were asked to assess which of the problems identified would have to be alleviated to restore a tolerable situation at home. Forty-six (92 per cent) were able to to this. The problems identified were divided into three groups:

1. Dependant's behaviour pattern

2. Supporter's own limitations
3. Environmental and social conditions
(See Tables 6.1, 6.2 and 6.3).

Of the difficulties supporters felt unable to cope with in the future home management, 80 per cent were in group 1, 11 per cent in group 2 and 9 per cent in group 3. The degrees of tolerance are well illustrated in the tables. Sleep disturbance and faecal incontinence were poorly tolerated in group 1 as might be expected, but surprisingly urinary incontinence and inability to wash and dress were coped with reasonably well. The important point is that when patients are nursed at home, a careful study has to be made of the factors most needing alleviation in the opinion of the helpers. Failure to recognise these can produce undue strain on families and although basic care may still be present, crisis may be imminent and urgent action is often necessary to support these helpers.

An acute social emergency arises when help ceases. This may be due to illness, either physical or mental in the helper, or when there are other commitments such as nursing a sick child or dealing with other family matters. Sometimes the helper has to move away from the area due to change in the spouse's occupation. Help may then stop altogether for an old person living alone. Even when a grandmother is living with the younger family, the arrival of a new baby may make it impossible, perhaps because of the shortage of space, for this to continue. The age of the helper may be important; sometimes the supplier of basic care is elderly herself and may be unable to continue carrying the burden. In all situations sometimes enough is enough; and particularly where a patient has mental illness, the carers can come to the end of their tether and demand help.

Cases are found when basic care is insufficient despite family presence in the area. Isaacs and his co-authors in the book *Survival of the Unfittest* examines 39 examples of this type in some detail.[5] The reasons why the social condition of old people was allowed to deteriorate despite the presence of available family were divided into four groups; preoccupation, dilemma, refusal and rejection. These will be discussed separately.

Preoccupation was considered to be the reason why 17 of the 39 patients with children in the area failed to receive adequate care and is a circumstance which will be well understood by anyone having to deal with old people. The relatives provided as much care as they could and

Table 6.1: Analysis of Group 1 Problems Identified (Dependants' Behaviour Patterns)

	Frequency (Percentage of Cases)	Tolerance (Percentage of Supporters Able to Tolerate Problems)
Sleep disturbance	62	16
Night wandering	24	24
Micturition	24	17
Shouting	10	20
Incontinence of faeces	56	43
Incontinence of urine	54	81
Falls	58	52
Inability to get out of bed unaided	52	35
Inability to get into bed unaided	50	40
Inability to get on commode unaided	36	22
Inability to get off commode unaided	38	21
Dangerous, irresponsible behaviour	32	38
Inability to walk unaided	18	33
Inability to walk at all	16	13
Personality conflicts	26	54
Physically aggressive behaviour	18	44
Inability to dress unaided	44	77
Inability to wash and/or shave unaided	54	93
Inability to communicate	16	50
Daytime wandering	12	33
Inability to manage stairs unaided	10	60
Inability to feed unaided	12	67
Blindness	2	0

Source: J.R.A. Sanford, 'Tolerance of Debility in Elderly Dependants by Supporters at Home: Its Significance for Hospital Practice', *British Medical Journal*, vol.3 (1975), pp.471-3.

were anxious to give more, but were prevented from doing so by prior commitments from which they were quite unable to free themselves, or by an impediment which they could not overcome. These causes included the health of the helper or care of another dependant.

Dilemma is where significant basic care is withheld because relatives, although capable and willing to give more help than they did, were

Table 6.2: Analysis of Group 2 Problems Identified (Supporters' Own Limitations)

	Frequency (Percentage of Cases)	Tolerance (Percentage of Supporters Able to Tolerate Problem)
Anxiety/depression	52	65
Personality conflicts	26	54
Insufficient strength for lifting	22	73
Rheumatoid/osteoarthritis	12	67
Back strain	8	100
Bronchitis	6	33
Embarrassment	4	0
Other	12	67

Source: Sanford, 'Tolerance of Debility in Elderly Dependants'.

Table 6.3: Analysis of Group 3 Problems Identified (Environmental and Social Conditions)

	Frequency (Percentage of Cases)	Tolerance (Percentage of Supporters Able to Tolerate Problem)
Restriction of social life	42	57
Inability to leave dependant for more than one hour	28	71
Stairs within accommodation	26	85
Financial disadvantage	4	0
Other	4	0

Source: Sanford, 'Tolerance of Debility in Elderly Dependants'.

forced to accept a different course in the interest of their own families. The dilemma of son and daughter in these circumstances is whether to give prior consideration to the needs of the parent or to those of their own family. Often an attempt was made to do both, but even so, the parents still received insufficient care. These situations are often full of anguish and feelings of guilt on the part of the offspring, and recriminations on the part of the old person. They are a rich source of family dispute and friction.

Refusal is where adequate care is absent because the old person is unwilling to receive it. In Isaacs' studies these were almost all men and they were usually of an aggressively independent type, attracting very little love towards themselves and tending not to give any either. These patients would not admit that they needed help and did not like to put themselves in a situation of being obliged to anyone else. They were often in dreadful social circumstances and even when discovered by social workers were extremely difficult to help.

Rejection is where the patient seems to have been rejected by his or her children. This rejection was difficult to understand on first impression, but after further inquiry reasons were often found. Sometimes there was a family quarrel which went back for years and the rejection might initially have been on the parental side. Examples included a daughter thought not to have made a suitable marriage and a son who in the past had gone against parental wishes. Maybe the parents were ashamed of some event in the lives of the children, as in the case of one son who had been in prison. Alcoholism in the parents or long-standing quarrels about money might drive children away. Second marriages sometimes caused problems. Initially, this might have seemed a good idea, but once one partner had become ill, the other one might feel aggrieved at having responsibilities of care after so short a time. Children may have disapproved of the second marriage and subsequently may have proved unwilling to share in the care of a stepmother or stepfather. First marriages never ran into this sort of difficulty.

Sometimes a problem in providing care for elderly people is that they do not like to be in another person's debt, even if these people are their own children. The presence of grandchildren is often good in overcoming these difficulties because of opportunities to reciprocate. If these are absent it might mean that the elderly couple become reluctant to ask for help and so a situation of neglect can arise.

Environmental Factors

These are usually associated with housing. There may be physical deterioration of a property and problems such as leaking roofs. Many old people live in properties which are in slum clearance areas and these tend to become neglected. Vermin are attracted and may migrate to inhabited dwellings, particularly if these are dirty and poorly maintained. These areas are also happy hunting grounds for vandals and the remaining inhabitants can be harassed and disturbed. Eviction may sometimes happen to old people when financial resources are low and these threats to deprive them of shelter can be extremely distressing. Old persons living with relatives may sometimes find themselves homeless when the family has to move to a smaller house with no spare room.

Co-operation Problems

Crisis situations may occur when there is a failure of communication between the caring services. This may particularly happen when a hospital fails to inform the community social and medical services of an old person's discharge. This is fortunately becoming rare because of the development of liaison between the hospital-based social and nursing services and those in the community. Liaison should also be very close between hospital doctors and general practitioners. Lack of co-ordination of activity between general practitioners and domiciliary social workers may be a cause of trouble these days. Clear demarcation of the duties of a doctor and social workers is sometimes not obvious and can only be overcome by person-to-person discussion about individual cases.

Social Help

With an ageing population social problems are going to increase. Isaacs *et al.*[5] highlight the problems neatly with their triangles of dependency theories. For patients dying at home, the greater the age of death, the longer the periods of dependency. Similarly, for patients in hospital, the longer the period spent in hospital before death, the longer was the period of dependency preceding admission. There is going to be more rather than less dependency in future in the community.

The resources of the Social Service Department in helping with these problems are described in Chapter 9 and it is not the intention of this book to describe in detail the social worker's role in helping the individual, the family and the community, but three principles of social help emerge from the above analysis of social difficulties.

1. A preventive approach is important to avoid problems and crises. Every effort must be made to foresee undue strain in those caring for old people so that possible 'crisis of care' situations can be avoided.
2. Flexibility is essential. Some crises are only short-term, but extensive help may be required to cope with them on a full-time

basis. Others may become persistent but may be alleviated by short interval care at critical points through the day. Welfare home accommodation may be necessary for long or short periods to help in these situations. The care given therefore needs to be appropriate to the needs.

3. Co-operation between social and medical workers is vital in both the hospital and community and in particular in handling a patient who is being transferred from one to the other.

Notes

1. Bernard Isaacs and Yvonne Neville, *The Measurement of Need in Old People* (Edinburgh, Scottish Home and Health Department, 1972).

2. Anne Barlow and David Matthews, 'Need for and Receipt of Domiciliary Social Services amongst the Elderly', unpublished DHSS discussion document (1978).

Audrey Hunt, *The Elderly at Home* (Office of Population Censuses and Surveys, Social Survey Division) (London, HMSO, 1978).

4. J.R.A. Sanford, 'Tolerance of Debility in Elderly Dependent by Supporters at Home', *British Medical Journal*, vol.3 (1975), pp.471-3.

5. B. Isaacs *et al.*, *Survival of the Unfittest* (London, Routledge and Kegan Paul, 1972).

Further Reading

Irene Gore, *The Generation Jigsaw* (London, George Allen and Unwin, 1977).

PART THREE: CONTEMPORARY SOLUTIONS

The story now changes from an analytical and descriptive account of old people in society to a more constructive examination of how patterns of care are developing. The next two chapters will concern themselves primarily with a clinic for the elderly, but initially some ideas as to why a new look needs to be taken at the provision of care for old people will be given, together with some fundamental aims which such care ought to achieve.

7 DEVELOPING PATTERNS OF CARE

In preceding chapters an account has been given of some of the problems which exist in providing care for old people in the community. In summary, they relate to the increased numbers of old people, difficulties with hospital and community services and the changing attitudes towards care of both families and the community. None of these are likely to change very much within the near future, apart from the actual number of old people; this is likely to increase and hence make the situation worse. It appears, therefore, that there will be an extra work-load and it will of necessity fall on the community services and in particular on the primary health and social care teams.

Until now the pattern of care given to old people, both socially and medically, has characteristically been crisis-orientated. It has also always been patient-, relative- or neighbour-initiated. The services have waited for a problem to occur and an attempt has then been made to alleviate it by direct action. This has classically been the doctor's pattern of working; he has usually waited for a call for help before taking action, although to be fair some doctors have also had a tradition of visiting old people regularly. Unfortunately, this has usually developed on an *ad hoc* basis, and the visits have often become unnecessary, sometimes evolving into purely social encounters. This is arguably no bad thing, and the lucky recipients of such visits have often benefited considerably, even though the doctor has performed no specific medical function. The interest shown and the contact created has been of value and in a sense the visit has been an unstructured doctor-initiated act. But it is often not the right people who are being seen regularly in this way and to visit all old people would be quite impossible. The average number of people over 75 years old on a list of 2,500 patients is 125. This would mean doing 30 calls every week in addition to other practice commitments. However, this *ad hoc* visiting has been the pattern of care for decades and clearly we need to take a new look at what needs to be done to bring methods of care up to date.

Fortunately, to help with this task, there has developed over the past decade a much better understanding of the natural history of old age and the characteristics of illness amongst the elderly in the community. The interrelationship between physical, mental and social causes of disability; the phenomenon of unreported need; the principle of effective health; the usual presence of multiple pathology and multiple symptomatology; and the sometimes uncharacteristic presentation of illness are all now well recognised. There is also the very important vicious circle effect. Many mental and physical problems in old age are relatively minor but given several of them, they can interact together to reduce effective health, often quite significantly. Recognition and treatment of these minor conditions may substantially contribute to overall functional well-being and ability.

Other characteristics of old age are also now recognised, including the distinction between 'young' old age (from 65 to 75 years) and 'old' old age (75 onwards). Chronological age may not match biological age and there is a great diversity between the health of different people of the same age. Ageing is a very fluid process and there are long periods of health and social stability interrupted by episodes of acute physical or environmental difficulty. These are often overcome and the old person returns again to a balanced equilibrium. Some problems become long-term and support is therefore necessary, but the nature and extent of this may also vary from time to time.

Special problems affecting old people are now also more fully understood; faulty diets and the risk of sub-nutrition, hypothermia, the increased risk of falls and problems with treatment are all now seen to be possible dangers. Certain groups are specially at risk to these types of problem. They include those living alone, those bedfast, the bereaved, the very old and those recently discharged from hospital. It is also now understood that old people need to be considered when planning community resources in a wider context and have special claims on housing, transport and social services.

Progress has therefore been made into the understanding of the needs of the elderly in the community and what will be required of the services in the future. In the community the health care given to old people is normal whole-person medicine dealing with the multifactoral problems which can arise; these may be physical or mental and often have social components. It is in this sense true general-practice medicine and not geriatric medicine. It can, however, be helped by partnership with the specialised geriatric service provided by the hospital team and both general practitioner and consultant in geriatric medicine need to work closely together. It is probably better, however, to look at the service given by the primary health care team as care of old people in the community, and that provided by the hospital as specialised geriatric care.

How will this care develop in the future? It seems that a new look needs to be taken. There are several reasons why this should be done urgently. Some of the points have already been made, but for the sake of clarity they will now be summarised.

Reasons for Taking a New Look at Community Care for Old People

1. The medical and social care of old people in the community, although often done well and in a dedicated way, has basically been unstructured and has failed to take into account recently acquired better understanding of the problem.

2. The number of old people in the community is going to increase and there will be consequent high demand on both medical and social services.

3. Because of the pressure on hospital geriatric departments, it is unlikely that they will be able to cope fully with any additional workload. It is necessary therefore that the community services should accept further responsibilities in caring for old people.

4. The shift in age balance within the population and the fact that the younger working generation will have to support a high number of elderly pensioners will for economic reasons make it imperative for old people to be kept active, healthy and self-supporting in the community. The caring services will have to be more positive in aiming to achieve this.

5. Another economic reason is that the scarce resources of experienced manpower and finance will have to be used as effectively as possible in the community and not wasted on providing unnecessary services, or too much administration.

6. Associated with the above reasons is the fact that as the ageing process is becoming more understood, it appears that certain problems are preventable. It is therefore necessary that a preventive programme should be built into the overall pattern of care.

7. The medical and social services have hitherto tended to work in isolation. A new look at co-operation between the two is essential.

8. The professional services need to adjust to the changing attitudes and expectations of both society and the family to the care of its elderly members. The responsibilities of each need redefining.

9. The relationship and communication between institutional care and domiciliary care needs to be improved and areas of co-operation defined.

10. All members of the community (including the professionals working in it) need to be educated about the responsibilities of caring for old people. The role of the family especially needs restating.

Overall Aims of Caring for Old People at Home

Arising out of the indications for a new look at community care for the elderly is the necessity to redefine the aims of such care. These, again, will be listed for clarity. They are orientated towards professional workers, both medical and social, and leave aside for the present what society's attitudes should be.

1. To establish an accurate diagnosis on which logical treatment and accurate prognosis can be based. This implies good day-to-day care of old people and effective management of acute situations.

2. To improve an old person's functional performance. Cure may not always be possible and it may be hard to treat multiple pathology, but an attempt should always be made to improve the patient's effective health.

3. To keep old people in their homes in an active and mobile state. They must remain part of the community, be outward-looking and accept responsibility for caring for themselves. In this sense the provision of care in itself is not the prime aim of the community workers, but rather the education and encouragement of old people to care for themselves. What is important is that an appropriate and adequate level of care is provided at the right time.

4. To foster a team approach to the provision of care. This should involve both health and social workers who should form a *community care team*. It has been said that a doctor and his team should be interested solely in the medical aspects of an old person and that the social worker need only concern herself with social problems. In practice, this is not so. It is impossible for a doctor not to become involved in the broader social aspects of a patient's life and he is inevitably interested in the general provisions of care – otherwise his medical treatment would often be of no avail. This has long been a principle of the practice of medicine and close liaison has always existed in the hospital between doctors, nurses and almoners. Social workers also know that in practice many of the problems they see have medical causes and implications, and co-ordination of activity is essential.

5. To recognise 'at risk' situations. Examples of these are patients living alone, the housefast, the over-75-year-olds, the bereaved and those recently discharged from hospital. Special care is needed for these people.

6. To have a preventive outlook towards care. Problems such as unreported need, vicious circle effects, malnutrition, hypothermia, drug misuse and many social problems are all preventable.

7. To undertake general surveillance and maintenance of those on long-term treatment.

8. To provide adequate rehabilitation and resettlement services, particularly for patients recently discharged from hospital.

9. To provide adequate care for the dying patients. People should be able to die in their own home if this is what they wish.

10. To reduce the defeated by increasing the defended in the community. This is based on Isaacs' theory of patients being either protected, defended or defeated (see page 77).

11. To establish a good relationship between the whole team caring for the elderly patients, particularly in creating a close partnership between those providing institutionalised and domiciliary care.

12. To establish clear guidelines for care which can usually be expected to be provided by the family and that which should be provided by the state.

Achievement of Aims

Some of these objectives are already being fulfilled very effectively. Medical care of acute illness and the day-to-day management of problems as they arise is probably better in the United Kingdom than anywhere in the world. This aspect of community care needs no rethinking, but the concept of extending overall care beyond merely providing acute services is in the main undeveloped. For example, teamwork between workers is only sporadic, and preventive activities are on the whole non-existent.

A new approach is thus required. A good way of achieving many of these aims is by running a clinic for the elderly, based on general practice. Here, prevention, rehabilitation, resettlement, maintenance and health education can all be co-ordinated and the team can be brought together. It is ideal if this can take place at a specific time but the principles underlying what will be described as a clinic can, nevertheless, be incorporated into routine practice and community work.

Outline of a Clinic for the Elderly

Before describing the detailed running of a clinic which will be done in the next chapter, some general principles underlying its conception will be discussed. The idea of a clinic for the elderly came out of a screening clinic to find unreported need. This was a preventive activity and screening is crucial in this respect. Although a clinic has other functions, its preventive function is central, and it is essential to be clear as to what this means.

Prevention can be of three types: *primary prevention*, which means the elimination of conditions that cause disease; *secondary prevention*, which is the identification in the community of subjects who are in good health, but who can be shown to have precursor states which lead to an increased chance of disease developing (for example, carcinoma *in situ* of the uterine cervix); and *tertiary prevention*, which is the early detection of established disease so that it can be treated quickly and effectively in order that deterioration and complications do not occur.[1]

Screening the elderly falls into this latter group. It does not mean searching for pre-symptomatic illness, but rather tries to find early established disease at a stage when it can be effectively treated. In addition, social as well as medical problems are usually sought for during a screen of elderly patients. A screen does not arise from the patient's request for advice, but is initiated by the doctor and an obligation is therefore placed on him to validate the exercise.

Problems to be Solved by Screening

Every screening process has as its aim the solution of a particular problem and this must always be clearly defined. When screening old people the problem to be solved is really in three parts. The underlying feature is the fact that old people tend not to report medical and social difficulty. This produces three problems: the presence of unmet need amongst the elderly; the vicious circle effect of several minor unreported conditions leading to reduced functional ability; and the very fact of why old people should fail to report need.

The solving of these problems is the aim of preventive screening clinics. Finding and treating unreported conditions, especially those of a minor nature, which might have cumulative effects, is not difficult, but the question of why old people fail to report illness and whether anything can be done to help this is a deeper consideration. Mention has already been made of some of the reasons why this should happen. There has, however, been no work undertaken to determine whether screening helps to overcome the fact of an unreported need. Screening clinics can hopefully help by educating old people about the available services and encouraging their use.

Indeed it is probable that future studies, because of this, will show an increased utilisation of medical and social services after screening. It will probably be too much to expect any significant reduction in the incidence of future acute medico-social problems, although some types should be preventable. Nevertheless, the aim should be to make these incidents capable of better management once they have occurred.

Validation

Validation of the first two aims of a clinic has been attempted. Many criteria have been used to test whether the stated objectives have been achieved but a successful screening exercise is usually expected to satisfy the following eight points:

1. The screening should be capable of being applied to a specific group in the population, and that group should be easily reached.

Elderly patient screening is certainly applied to a specific group in the population. They can be easily identified using an age sex register of old people.

2. The screening process must be clear, easily repeatable, well defined, safe and reliable.
The procedure is quite clear cut. It consists of a health visitor interview and a doctor's examination, followed by any necessary action.

3. It should be practical on a large scale.
Screening old people is certainly practical in general practice and could be carried out widely. An average list of 2,500 patients would contain about 125 patients over 75. It would take only a year to see these patients at the rate of two per week.

4. It should be cheap.
The low cost to the community if it is carried out in general practice is self-evident.

5. It must be acceptable to patients.
Most surveys carried out in general practice have shown that the patients accept the procedure and even welcome it. The view is often expressed that old patients feel reassured after a full examination as a result of the screen.

6. It must have a satisfactory yield.
Most surveys have shown a high yield of morbid conditions and often the need for social services. The large number of patients needing some type of treatment is frequently commented upon by anyone undertaking this type of work. The yield expected from this type of

clinic therefore can be quite considerable.

7. The conditions isolated at screening should be capable of being effectively treated.
Unfortunately, very few follow-up studies have been done on patients screened at geriatric clinics. Lowther *et al.* evaluated their early diagnostic services for the elderly.[2] They found clear evidence of improvement in half of their patients who had carried out recommendations. If all patients examined were included, the proportion helped was about 23 per cent. Williams found similar figures in his follow-up.[3] Unfortunately, neither reviewed the minor conditions but experience in practice does seem to indicate that many of these are very treatable and when this is undertaken, improvement in function is achieved.

8. Does the screening process contribute to the recognition of unreported need and can this be shown to be so by looking at the group studied before and after the exercise?
Undoubtedly screening recognises unreported need and both Williams and Lowther found this in their original and follow-up studies. Lowther points out that early detection reduces the period of suffering in many conditions and avoids hospital admission. He states that some merit lies in the mere identification of disease. Unless a diagnosis is made, there can be no rational therapy and the questions of prevention can never arise. Whether screening is the answer to the whole problem of unreported need is not clear. No studies have been undertaken on screened and unscreened groups and no attempt has been made to determine if the exercise helps to make unreported need less common. These are tasks for the future.

The Advantages of Running a Clinic for the Elderly

When outlining the aims of good care for elderly people in the community, it was clear that, alongside efficient care of acute problems, must go adequate maintenance, proper rehabilitation and resettlement, a preventive outlook and education of patients and families. A team approach to these features of care was thought to be essential. A clinic for the elderly provides a focus where all these can be achieved as well as a place where problems can be discussed and smoothed out. From the clinic a more positive commitment to keeping old people at home can be made and skilled resources used more effectively. Above all, an outlook that aims to keep old people active and functionally sound can be fostered.

Doctors and members of the team can also learn from the old people. Insight into the nature of old age, the natural history of illness and the problems and joys of these patients can readily be gained during screening sessions. The long and interesting lives of these old people are sometimes overlooked if contact is restricted to dealing only with acute crisis situations.

Dangers

Perhaps in outlining concepts of care in the way that has been done in this chapter, there is the risk of appearing too idealistic. Problems do, however, exist, and although it is realised that a great deal of what has been advocated goes on already during normal medical practice, much that can be done, nevertheless, goes by default. Enthusiasm is necessary but can bring dangers. There is a risk of over-treatment and this is discussed in Chapter 12. A patient's life can be made more difficult by being given too many drugs. It is also possible to make a patient aware of problems which had previously caused him little trouble. It would be wrong to upset a patient's equilibrium by drawing attention to these and it might be well just to note them and say nothing. As with all screening examinations, it is vital that negative cases should in fact be negative. It would be disastrous to miss something important and reassure the patient that all was well, and that he failed to report subsequent symptoms because of this. It is essential that screening should be thorough.

Another criticism levelled at screening clinics is that they may make the doctor and his team complacent. Once seen at a clinic there may be danger of the old person being forgotten. This is unlikely. If difficulties exist surveillance is usually instituted; if all is well, education and instruction will have been given to encourage the patient to report back.

Some doctors and members of the primary health care team assert that they already know all their elderly patients and screening is unnecessary. Yet it is surprising how often somebody is brought to a clinic who has not been seen for some time, despite having been collecting repeat prescriptions, and who was obviously long overdue for review.

Notes

1. James Williamson, 'Preventive Aspects of Geriatric Medicine', *Modern Geriatrics*, vol.1, no.1 (1970), p.24.

2. C.P. Lowther, R.D.M. Macleaod and J. Williamson, 'Evaluation of Early Diagnostic Services for the Elderly', *British Medical Journal*, vol.3 (1970), pp.275-7.

3. E.I. Williams, 'A Follow-up of Geriatric Patients after Sociomedical Assessment', *Journal of the Royal College of General Practitioners*, vol.24 (1974), pp.341-6.

Further Reading

J. Williamson, 'Detecting Disease in Clinical Geriatrics', *Gerontologia Clinica*, vol.9 (1967), pp.236-42.

Sir W. Ferguson Anderson, 'The Effect of Screening on the Quality of Life after 70' *Journal of the Royal College of General Practitioners*, vol.10, no.2 (1976).

8 A CLINIC FOR THE ELDERLY

When setting up a clinic for the elderly, the first step will usually be to organise a screening exercise. This enables patients to be reviewed, possible problems to be forecast and 'at risk' groups to be identified. The first part of this chapter will describe in some detail the running of such a screening exercise, and later the other functions of a clinic for the elderly will be described.

Organisation of Clinic

Age/Sex Register

The first essential is to form an Age/Sex register for the elderly. This can be done with the help of the Family Practitioner Committee for patients of 65 years and over. Details of the patient's name, address, date of birth, sex and, if known, occupation, are included on small cards which are stored in a standard metal filing cabinet (the Royal College of General Practitioners provides cards which are suitable for use in an Age/Sex register). These cards are kept in birthday order, the males being separated from the females. When the list is first obtained from the Family Practitioner Committee, it is usual to compare details with the practice notes. Occasionally, patients have died or moved to a new address and records need updating. An early task is to feed into the system details of patients who are in hospital, welfare homes or nursing homes. Some research practices have their Age/Sex registers linked to a computer, but in normal practice work this is unnecessary. Having established the register, the task of keeping it up to date should be given to one member of the practice staff.

Age of Entry into Screen

There is a difference of opinion as to what is the correct age to start screening. It has been said that the real problems of old age start at around the age of 75 and it is above this age that screening becomes productive. Certainly, younger old people retain the ability to report problems. Probably the best age to include patients in the screening exercise is about 72, although this is quite arbitrary and any age between then and 75 would be suitable. An attempt should be made to see all patients over the chosen age. This in the first place will need spreading over a couple of years, but once completed, only those reaching the appropriate birthday and those on periodic review will need to be seen. The numbers are going to increase, but at present it would involve seeing about 7 per cent of the total practice list, or 175 patients from an average list of 2,500.

Who Does the Screen?

By far the best combination is that of a doctor and health visitor with a social worker involved if this is possible. It has been said that health visitors can screen old people themselves by asking selected questions and looking for certain important clinical signs. Perhaps most significant medical conditions can be found in this way and referred to the doctor, but many of the unreported problems of old people are relatively minor and full examination is often necessary to discover these. Doctor examination is undoubtedly valuable as it gives the patient confidence, and treatment, referral and investigation can be immediately arranged. If this is impossible, obviously health visitor screening is useful; but ideally, the exercise is one of teamwork and should involve all the members of the practice.

Invitation to the Patient

In early screening exercises this was done by a letter of invitation explaining the nature of the exercise and asking for co-operation. Enclosed was a prepaid reply card on which the patients were asked if they agreed to co-operate and whether they were able to come to the surgery themselves, needed transport or whether their condition necessitated a visit from the doctor at home. These early reply cards worked very well and produced a response rate of up to 85 per cent, but they could be criticised on several grounds. It was not easy to explain in a letter the exact nature of the screen and the preventive aspects of it. It was difficult for some, particularly very old patients, to understand why the doctor wanted to see them and a few questioned his motives. Invitation by letter can also be criticised on the grounds that a screen could take place without anyone being aware of what the home and environmental circumstances might be. It therefore seemed essential to include some kind of assessment of the patient's actual living conditions. For these reasons, it is probably better if patients are visited by the health visitor and asked if they will participate in the screening exercise. During this invitation visit, an assessment of the housing situation can be made. This method, although more time-consuming, has increased the response in some screens to 100 per cent and has also enabled more realistic transport arrangements to be made. It is therefore the method to be recommended.

Transport

This may present certain problems, as transporting patients to general practitioners' surgeries or health centres is not included in the NHS provisions. Sometimes volunteers can be recruited to transport old people to the surgery. It might also be possible for the health visitor or member of the practice staff to undertake the task, providing insurance cover is adequate. In the author's original screening sessions, those people who were unable to make their own way to the surgery were brought by car by volunteers. These car drivers were often young mothers recruited from the practice, who added a touch of brightness to the lives of the old folk and often permanent friendships were formed.

In some areas there are pilot schemes using ambulances to transport old people to clinics and this might become more widespread in the future.

Pro Formas

It is useful to have standard check-lists or pro formas for the screen which can be incorporated into the practice notes. These provide a good base line for any future medical or social incident. The format of a check-list does, however, provide problems. The present record system consists of envelopes which are totally inadequate to incorporate any volume of information. Either only a small amount of detail is recorded or an attempt must be made to convert the whole of the over-65 record system to A4 size. This is DHSS policy and its implementation will certainly make it easier to run screening clinics. Perhaps the local Family Practitioner Committees should assist financially in this changeover. Another difficulty is to know how detailed to make the assessment of the old person and hence the pro forma. Many examples have been produced, but it is possibly best for the doctor and health visitor to work out their own schemes.[1,2] In general, these will be in three sections: the health visitor interview, the doctor examination and a final assessment of action and follow-up plans. These three parts of the screening process will now be examined in a little detail.

Health Visitor Interview

Note on History-Taking in Old People

There are difficulties in taking a history from an old person. The memory may be failing, deafness may be present and complaints may not be precise. Sometimes for these reasons the old patients fail to give a reasonable account of themselves and when faced with a health visitor or doctor, may still overlook significant symptoms, although some may do better with the health visitor than the doctor. It is therefore useful to have a relative present at a screening clinic, so that information may be confirmed and supplemented. The medical history is often very long and much of it is irrelevant. Considerable discernment is necessary to identify what is important, particularly when the patient is an enthusiastic raconteur. Illness sometimes progresses at different rates in old people and this must be remembered when interpreting symptoms. The fact that a symptom may have been present for some time may not necessarily rule out serious illness. For example, an old person may discount ankle swelling and breathlessness because its development has been insidious. Chronic symptoms may have come to be accepted and disregarded, whereas those which have only just developed within the last few days are given prominence. Different significance is sometimes placed on symptoms by old people; thus, tiredness, which may be due to iron deficiency anaemia, may be ignored. Some symptoms, on the other hand, such as tinnitus or itching are very distressing and complained of readily. Nevertheless, what is important to the health visitor may not be so to the patient. For these reasons, direct questioning is very necessary to elicit vital information.

General Information

Obviously, the name, address, sex, date of birth, marital status, occupation (or that of the spouse) need to be recorded, but it is also useful to know the name and address of the next of kin and any relevant telephone numbers. It is also interesting to note when the patient last visited the doctor. Height and weight should also be recorded.

Social Assessment

If a social worker is included in the team, a full professional social assessment may be made. Failing this, it is nevertheless possible and necessary to elicit certain important social information. The idea is to assess the general suitability of the patient's environment and his ability to cope with looking after himself within it. It is necessary to know whether the patient lives alone, is housefast, or bedfast. If he does live alone, note should be made of how long he has done so and what support he has from, and contact he has with, relatives, friends and neighbours. If not living alone, the state of health and composition of other members of the household may be relevant. Capacity for self-care can be assessed by ability to wash, dress, toilet, cook and do the housework. Ability to undertake shopping, social activities and hobbies should also be noted. The suitability of the dwelling is also important; it may be a house or flat, rented or owned, and details of the number of rooms and adequacy of the washing, toileting and cooking facilities should be noted. Assessment of heating, ventilation and any possible accident hazards is necessary. Finally, the general state of the repair of the house should be observed.

Diet

An account of the nutritional state of old people is given in Chapter 17. During the screen it is essential to determine whether an old person is taking an adequate diet. Some direct questions are usually necessary and the minimum aim should be for him to have one cooked meal per day.

Finance

It is not easy to raise directly with people the question of financial difficulty. Many do not receive their full entitlement of allowances, and it may be necessary to give advice about these. Sometimes the person is financially secure but he is reluctant to spend money on obviously needed items such as clothes, shoes, extra heating and food. Patients occasionally need to be gently persuaded by the health visitor to spend a little of their savings.

Previous Medical Treatment

A note may be made of any significant previous illness, injury and operation.

Current Medical Treatment

The treatment that a patient is receiving at the time of the screen needs tabulating so that it can be reviewed and entered on a co-operation card. It is often interesting to find out in addition what he is taking in the way of self-medication.

Doctor Examination

Note on Examining Old People

The first essential when examining an old person is to make him or her feel comfortable and relaxed. The room should be warm and the examination couch fixed at such a level that the patient can get on and off easily. The back rest should be at an appropriately high angle, as many old people cannot lie flat. Undressing sometimes presents a problem and the health visitor or practice nurse can help with this. Occasionally an old person will refuse to undress and then it will be necessary to use ingenuity and the 'keyhole' technique where small areas of body are exposed progressively through gaps in clothing. Many physical changes take place with ageing, and should be taken into account when conducting an examination.

Assessment of General Condition

Much can be learnt about the patient by merely observing his appearance and behaviour. He may be clean and smartly dressed or untidy with food-stained clothes, indicating a lack of interest or deteriorating ability for self-care. Watching someone move and climb on to the couch may indicate that he has problems with mobility. The patient's face may display emotions of worry and anxiety or alternatively he may appear happy and contented. How well an old man has shaved or whether an old lady still uses make-up may give a clue as to how much self-interest is retained and also whether good manual dexterity is still present. Speech may show defects such as slurring or change in pitch. Note should be made of any recent weight loss, and the temperature, using a low-reading thermometer, should also be taken.

Mental State

General mental alertness and whether the patient is bright and cheerful should be noted. Simple tests such as asking him to recall the name of the Prime Minister or even more personal facts like his own birthday, or home address, can be carried out to determine memory deficiency and inadequate orientation. Early dementias can be recognised in this way. Psychotic illness may also be present and need diagnosing. A knowledge of the patient's previous personality can be helpful in this respect. For instance, if a previously well-dressed professional man presents a picture of untidiness and lack of personal hygiene, it could indicate the presence of early mental deterioration.

Mobility

Mobility needs assessing on a functional basis, testing, for instance, whether a patient is able to walk, stand, and particularly whether he can do this without loss of balance. Any unsteadiness or restriction of movement can be due to a variety of skeletal and neurological conditions. Examination of both these systems when mobility is being assessed is helpful. Examination of the feet is also important.

Evidence of Anaemia

Anaemia is common in old people and routine blood testing is essential; but it is nevertheless interesting, during clinical examination, to make an assessment of the possibility and degree of anaemia. During an examination of nearly 300 patients by the author, an assessment of anaemia was attempted, using as guides the colour of the conjunctiva and the condition of the skin, finger-nails and tongue (Williams and Nixon).[3] The mean haemoglobin level of those showing evidence of anaemia clinically was calculated and compared with the remainder of the group. Evidence of anaemia judged by pallor of the conjunctivae was found to be the best guide.

Endocrine System

Most of the endocrine diseases occurring in old age are treatable. Diabetes may be suspected from the history, but it is usually diagnosed by urine and blood testing. Thyroid and adrenal disorders need careful assessment, as there is sometimes a fine line between changes due to old age itself and those due to disease.

Alimentary Tract

Examination of the digestive system starts with a look at the teeth. Not all old people are edentulous and some have a good set of teeth. These may, however, need treatment and the aim should be to preserve them for as long as possible. Many old people have ill-fitting dentures which they have possessed for many years. Whether these should be replaced rather depends on how the patient is managing. Dental advice is usually necessary. Further examination of the alimentary tract proceeds in the normal way, with a special look at the hernial orifices as hernia is not uncommon.

Possible pitfalls are an enlarged liver, due to distortion of the thoracic cage, a pulsating aorta which is often felt in old people, and does not necessarily imply an aneurysm, and lumps of hard faeces which are present in the descending colon. Rectal examination also often reveals problems, for instance haemorrhoids, fistulas and skin lesions. A small, hard prostate may be present and signify neoplasm.

Genito-urinary Tract

It is important to recognise overflow incontinence and bladder distension may be present without the patient being aware of it. Gynaecological conditions such as prolapse and vulval abnormality are not uncommon.

Cardiovascular System

A complete examination of the cardiovascular system is necessary as many incipient problems may be found. Interpretation of the findings, however, is often difficult. Wide variations are found in, for instance, blood pressure levels. If the blood pressure has been taken in both arms and differences of more than 20mm Hg is found, it may suggest disease of the inter-thoracic arterial system. Arteriosclerosis is often seen and when the arm is bent at the elbow, the so-called locomotor brachialis sign of the beating radial artery can be observed. Arrhythmias and signs of heart failure should be noted and also the condition of the peripheral pulses together with the presence or absence of oedema.

Respiratory System

Examination of the respiratory system is along normal lines, remembering the changes in respiratory function in old age. Attention can also be paid to the breasts during examination of the chest with a special watch for any signs of neoplasm.

Eyesight

Visual acuity can be measured by simple functional tests. For instance, an idea of the efficiency of a patient's eyesight can be found by asking whether he is able to watch television, read a newspaper, and assessed by seeing if he can read print at a short distance. Visual fields should also be tested and an examination of the fundi, lenses and pupil reflexes undertaken as a routine.

Hearing

Hearing can again be measured by simple functional tests such as whether the patient is capable of hearing a shouted or whispered voice.

Hearing aids, if worn, should also be tested for their efficiency, and the ears should be examined by auriscope to check for wax.

Skin

The natural changes in the skin due to ageing are discussed elsewhere. Many conditions are, however, often present which need treatment or point to general disease. Evidence of injury, bruising, ulceration, burns or dermatitis are examples. Signs of vitamin C deficiency can also be detected by examination of the skin and the mucous membranes of the mouth. Rodent ulcers on the face should be noted, and treatment, so successful these days, arranged.

Urine Testing

Is it worth testing the urine of patients seen at screening clinics? During the survey undertaken in 1972 of patients over 75 years of age, by the author and co-workers, 272 specimens of urine were examined, of which 6 were found to contain albumen and 10 to contain sugar.[4] Eight of these patients with sugar in the urine were not known to be diabetic and 5 resulted in a diagnosis of diabetes mellitus. Most of the patients found to have albumen in their urine were women. One was a man who was found to be suffering from a urinary infection. Using Lab stix methods, the presence of ketones and blood can also be determined. Assessing the significance of positive findings in the urine is sometimes difficult and usually further investigation is necessary. Glycosuria has several possible causes and proteinuria, although often associated with infection, may be caused by more serious renal and extra renal disease.

Blood Tests

It is desirable when screening an old person to undertake a haematological assessment. The possible range of tests is wide. Which to undertake should be made on a common-sense basis, and pathologist consultation is necessary to determine which is locally practicable. On a pragmatic basis it may be that haemoglobin, film, urea and sugar are the investigations which bring most in the way of practical return. However, a full list would probably include:

Haemoglobin
FBC and film
ESR or plasma viscosity
Blood sugar
Blood urea and electrolytes (sodium and potassium)

Chemical profile (calcium, phosphorus, alkaline phosphatase, bilirubin, LDH and transaminase)
T_4, T_3 uptake and Free thyroid index
Serum lipids
Serum proteins and possibly electrophoresis
Acid phosphatase
Serum folate and B_{12}

The volume of blood to be taken and the bottles required need also to be arranged with the Pathological Department, but will usually be in the region of 20ml. Fixing of normal parameters will again have to be determined in consultation with the pathologist undertaking the tests.

Assessment and Action

When the health visitor interview and the doctor examination are complete, an assessment consultation is necessary to consider the findings and plan future action. This usually involves the doctor and health visitor but could also involve a social worker and the community nursing sister. The assessment has five main parts:

1. to construct a list of the medical and social disabilities found;
2. to assess the patient's effective health;
3. to prepare action charts and initiate any necessary arrangements and treatment (see Table 8.1);
4. to make follow-up arrangements;
5. to issue co-operation cards.

These will now be discussed in more detail.

1. Abnormalities Found

A list of the medical disabilities and social problems need to be compiled. Some of the diagnoses and problems may perhaps need to be provisional, pending further investigation and consultation. It is interesting to note whether the conditions were already known to the practice or whether they were unreported.

2. Effective Health

In Chapter 3 the concept of effective health was discussed and a definition given of the main groups. It can be a helpful indicator of the usefulness of the screen to note whether the effective health of the old person has been changed as a result of the intervention.

Table 8.1: A Clinic for the Elderly: Action Possibilities Following Geriatric Screening

General Action List	
1. Nothing	8. Nursing services
2. Note of at risk situations	9. Chiropody
3. Treatment	10. Physiotherapy
4. Health visitor surveillance	11. Occupational therapy
5. Social services	12. Optician
6. Use of hospital services	13. Dentist
7. Investigation	14. Voluntary services
Social Service Possibilities	
1. Rehousing	8. Day centre
2. Home help	9. Additional heat
3. Luncheon club	10. Social casework
4. Welfare home	11. Laundry
5. Meals on wheels	12. Appliances
6. Holiday relief	13. Financial aid
7. Blind register	14. Mental health advice

3. Action

The action possibilities are as follows.

(1) Nothing. The first possibility is that the patient requires no services, no treatment and no investigation. This occurred in about one-third of the patients in the survey undertaken by the author, and this is probably the sort of figure which can be generally expected. The fact that no action is needed does not mean, however, that the patient has not benefited from the screen. Very often during the course of the interview and examination small points are discussed and advice given. These are not necessarily noted as action required. It is possible that most old people receive some general advice. There is also the more subtle benefit that is derived from the patient merely gaining contact with the medical and social services and being reassured that nothing is wrong. It is useful for a patient to be told the correct procedure for contacting the doctor in an emergency and to know how an appointment can be made. A card with the telephone number of the practice can be given. He may also be introduced to other members of the practice staff and realise that he can have direct access to the health

visitor. This is all part of the health education function of the clinic.

(2) Note of 'at risk' situations. Special note needs taking of any problems of diet, finance, accident hazards (including possibility of falls in the house) and difficulties with retirement, work or re-employment. A review of the drugs currently being taken also needs to be made. Special 'at risk' patients will be recognised at this point.

(3) Treatment. Specific treatment often needs to be given for conditions found and perhaps the therapy which the patient is already receiving needs adjustment. The basic principles of drug treatment in old age are outlined in Chapter 12.

(4) Health Visitor Surveillance. Apart from being involved in the clinic, the health visitor has many other roles to perform when looking after old people. The range of her services is extensive and includes health teaching, direct provision of care and support, follow-up surveillance and liaison with other agencies. She will be interested in social as well as medical problems and will be involved in arranging for any necessary social services if a social worker is not available. Follow-up visits may be needed and often discussion with the patient's family. The help of voluntary organisations can be arranged by the health visitor.

(5) Social Services. These are listed in Table 8.1 and discussed more fully in Chapter 9.

(6) Use of Hospital Services. Hospital admission may sometimes be necessary for the treatment of some acute condition found at the clinic. This is usually to an acute medical/geriatric ward but may also involve ENT ophthalmic or psychiatric departments. Admission may be also necessary to geriatric departments for further investigation and particularly for rehabilitation. Occasionally, it might be obvious that an old person is in need of long-stay hospital care. Hospital out-patient referral may be necessary and may involve the full range of specialist care (apart of course from the paediatric and maternity departments!). Domiciliary consultations by hospital consultants are very useful if the patient is housefast or bedfast. Day hospital care may be appropriate and the advice of the consultant geriatrician is important in assessing this type of case. In some areas there is a half-way house system, where the GP has access to beds in a general hospital or more usually in a community hospital.

Surgical treatment. The possibilities of surgical treatment in old people have now much improved. It is only in extreme old age that the GP is faced with the problem of whether or not surgery is realistic. Modern techniques now make it feasible to operate on extremely old people in emergencies. Thus, a patient suffering from acute appendicitis or intestinal obstruction should be referred directly to the surgeon. Patients suffering from fractures, particularly of the femur, are treated routinely by plating or hip replacement.

A more difficult problem arises when the patient suffers from a carcinoma in late old age. Whether or not to treat is dependent to some extent on his general condition, but even so, surgical opinion should be sought as palliative measures might become necessary and the surgeon should be involved at an early stage.

(7) Investigation. A full range of medical investigation is available to old people and should be used if there is any question of doubt about the diagnosis. Further blood testing, urine analysis and X-rays are easily arranged but more complicated procedures will usually involve referral to hospital consultants.

(8) Nursing Services. The help of both the practice nurse and the domiciliary nursing team may be needed following screening. The role of nursing care for old people is discussed in Chapter 10.

(9) Chiropody. Arrangements can be made in the clinic for a patient to visit a chiropodist or for treatment to be given at home. This may even be restricted to a simple nail-cutting and foot hygiene service. Most Area Health Authorities have a chiropody service available for old people.

(10) Physiotherapy. A full account of the role of physiotherapy is described in Chapter 11 on rehabilitation. Physiotherapy may be arranged through the hospital or in areas where it exists through domiciliary physiotherapy services.

(11) Occupational Therapy. Again, this is discussed in the chapter on rehabilitation. It is usually arranged through the hospital and is particularly suitable for day hospital care. Some local authorities have occupational therapy services associated with the provision of aids and appliances. Help is available from them in assessing needs and training in the use of aids.

(12) Optician. The services of the NHS opticians are fully available to old people and eye testing can be arranged at screening clinics. If vision is severely affected, the advice of a consultant ophthalmologist is required. Full discussion of these problems takes place in Chapter 17.

(13) Dentists. Old people sometimes require dental services either for attention to their own teeth or renewal and adjustment of dentures. Occasionally, it is necessary to arrange for a domiciliary visit to a patient's home.

(14) Voluntary Services. The help of volunteers is sometimes vital in arranging for the care of old people. Local 'good neighbour' schemes are to be encouraged and also help with transport, shopping, etc. Many organisations exist to help with this type of work and usually the health visitor will be aware of the help available locally.

4. Follow-up Arrangements

Follow-up arrangements are important but must be flexible. They are determined by the patient's needs and condition. Sometimes maintenance necessitates continuous supervision, whereas if the patient is in good effective health and not on treatment, there is probably no need for routine examination for maybe three years unless a new situation develops.

Identified 'at risk' groups need following up at specific intervals, usually by the health visitor or community nursing services. Some patients will have to be reviewed a month after screening to see whether treatment has been carried out and whether services have been provided. This type of review can often be undertaken by the health visitor.

5. Co-operation Card

It is usual at the conclusion of the screen to issue the patient with a card showing the current treatment. This can be carried around by the patient and be available to provide information to other doctors and paramedical workers who might be subsequently involved in management.

Other Functions of the Clinic

Health Maintenance

Ageing is a continuing process and situations can change. It is impossible to undertake complete surveillance of every patient, but some 'at risk' people can be singled out for regular contact with some member of the team. These patients would include those living alone, the housefast, the recently bereaved, and those vulnerable to poor diet, hypothermia and falls. In old age, health maintenance really means keeping an old person functionally independent and a watch must be kept not only on his physical and mental condition but also his social and environmental state. Patients with specific diseases demanding continuing care could be seen regularly at a clinic. Sometimes the need for treatment or services changes and it is occasionally necessary to discontinue some of these.

Resettlement

A particular situation which can be managed from a clinic for the elderly is when a patient is discharged from hospital. Co-operation between the hospital staff, the practice nursing team, the domiciliary social worker and the health visitor in ensuring continued care, especially with rehabilitation, can be facilitated if it is known that these workers meet at a specific time each week at the health centre or practice surgery. It is useful for the practice secretary to be informed of discharge from hospital of old people so that she can alert the team.

Health Education

Educating old people, their families and neighbours about the general principles of health care for the elderly can be arranged through the clinic, with the health visitor playing a prominent role.

Other Preventative Measures

Primary prevention may also be undertaken at clinics for the elderly and a good example of this is immunisation against influenza. There may be other developments along these lines in the future.

Direct Referral

Sometimes a patient seen during a surgery or on a home visit needs further investigation. It is often possible to refer them to the clinic for full assessment. Again, relations may contact the doctor and express concern about an old person. It is very useful to be able to refer somebody, brought to the doctor's attention in this way, to the clinic for review.

Notes

1. I.H. Stokoe, 'Care of the Elderly', *Update* Plus (1971), pp.677-84.
2. J.M. Tomlinson, 'Setting up a Geriatric Survey in General Practice', *Update*, vol.12, no.3 (1976), pp.277-88.
3. E.I. Williams and J.V. Nixon, 'Haemoglobin Levels in a Group of 75-year-old Patients in General Practice', *Gerontologica Clinica*, vol.16 (1974), pp.210-18.
4. E.I. Williams *et al.*, 'Sociomedical Study of Patients over 75 in General Practice', *British Medical Journal*, vol.2 (1972), pp.445-8.

PART FOUR: RESOURCES AVAILABLE IN THE COMMUNITY

There are resources available in the community to the team providing overall care. These can be utilised during an acute episode of illness or social breakdown, but can also be available at a clinic for the elderly. Four important resource activities are described in this section. Each is primarily the responsibility of one member of the team, but each should be aware of the role of the others.

9 SOCIAL RESOURCES IN THE COMMUNITY

Most advanced countries have community welfare services but they sometimes differ in form and emphasis. Many European countries, such as Denmark and Sweden, have a long history of social care of old people, and a wide variety of service is now available. In the USA such care was started much later and was mainly centred on institutions. Self-help has always been a strong life philosophy in the USA but recently community-based services have been developed to help the aged. In Russia, a full range of services is provided with particular emphasis on prevention of problems and rehabilitation of old people back into the community. In the UK a very comprehensive service is provided for old people. Help is available from Local Authorities through the Social Service and Housing Departments. Financial help is available from central government through the Department of Health and Social Security. In addition to this, a considerable amount of assistance is given by voluntary and religious organisations.

Social Services

The provision of social help for needy old people has been established in the UK for a considerable time as part of the package available under the old Poor Law provisions. Since the Second World War it has been consistent government policy to enable old people to continue living at home for as long as possible and to this end legislation has been passed to enable Local Authorities to provide supporting services. The National Assistance Act of 1948 required Local Authorities to provide residential accommodation for persons who by reasons of age, infirmity or any other circumstance are in need of care and attention which is not otherwise available to them. The Chronically Sick and Disabled Persons Act of 1970 and Section 45 of the Public Health Services Act of 1968 gave Local Authorities power to act to help old people in the community. The Local Authority Social Services Act of 1970 formalised many of the services being provided, and brought into being the unified Local Authority Social Services Department.

The newly formed Social Service Departments have been particularly interested in promoting the welfare of old people, although they have encountered many difficulties, not the least of which was the further reorganisation of local government which brought new authorities into being on 1 April 1974. The resulting redistribution of boundaries should reduce some of the difficulties and where these happen to be coterminous with those of Area or District Health Authorities, better co-operation may be achieved. There has, however, been a further problem of finance and manpower availability and this has not yet been resolved.

Despite these difficulties, certain aims and philosophies have been developed by the various departments. It is emerging that the primary concern of social work is not so much the provision of services, but more to recognise social problems. By doing this, it is hoped that intervention by a professional worker will make it possible to bring about changes which will enable the problem, once recognised, to be resolved, and hence enable the family to remain independently in the community and function without support. If this fails, it will then be necessary to provide ongoing support services and so once more enable the person to lead as full and satisfying life as possible. A further objective is to try to prevent social distress notably by early intervention, but also by preventive measures, using community work skills.

The range of possible services will now be described. Information about these is available locally; or can be obtained centrally in England and Wales from the Department of Health and Social Security and in Scotland from the Social Work Department of the Scottish Office.

Home Help

Over half a million elderly people received assistance from the Home Help Service in the year ending March 1976. The service enables an old person to receive help in the house of a domestic nature and it usually involves 2-3 hours per day for any number of days in the week. The duties of a home help are general cleaning and tidying, but can also include some cooking and shopping. It is the intention that the home help should do some of the heavier work which is beyond the ability of the old person. The visit can also provide interest and company which relieves loneliness and acts as a contact with the outside world, and particularly with the Social Services Department. The extent of the Home Help services provided by Local Authorities is limited and is not enough in general to satisfy the needs of the population. The financial arrangements vary from place to place. Some Authorities provide a free service on the grounds that the deserving will not then be afraid to ask. Other Authorities make a charge based on a means test and the person's resources are assessed at the same time as the need for assistance by the local home help organiser. Occasionally, emergency home help teams are available when crisis situations develop and urgent provision of help is necessary.

Meals on Wheels

The elderly are the principal receivers of meals on wheels and in the year ending March 1976, just under 24.5 million meals were taken to old people's homes and almost 170,000 elderly people were helped in this way. Over half of the meals taken to homes were delivered by members of voluntary organisations, notably the WRVS. The old person is usually provided with a hot midday meal on two or three days of the week. This is usually not quite enough to meet the requirement. The nutritional value of the meal is good and although the old person has to pay, the service is subsidised by the Local Authority. In some areas the extent of the service is widened to provide meals at other times of the day and at weekends. Emergency meals on wheels are also sometimes available.

Luncheon Clubs

This is an extension of the meals on wheels service. Luncheons are provided at centres often located in community homes or church halls. The service is principally used by old people sufficiently mobile to make their own way there. It enables the old person to get out of the house and become involved in a little social activity. It has the advantage of efficiency, so that more old people can be catered for. The meal is supervised by a responsible person who, as a secondary objective, can keep an eye on the group and detect any signs of deterioration or increasing inability to cope.

Day Centres/Day Care

These are really of two types. A day centre may merely be a meeting place where old people can attend to see old friends and engage in social activities. Hobbies may be catered for and there may be the opportunity for games and craft work. Sometimes the centre is in the form of a workshop where old people can come for certain hours during the day, to work and earn a little money.

A different type of centre is where day care is provided. Here full residential care is available in the day time and the centre is often associated with a residential home. Full supervision is present and meals are given. The type of person attending these is usually dependent on some sort of care, particularly if he or she lives alone or the family is unable to provide care throughout the day. Transport is often provided for old people to get to and from the centre. This type of care is also useful in providing an intermediate stage between residential accommodation and return to a person's own home. It also may mark an intermediate stage between a patient living at home and entering full-time residential accommodation. It allows more flexibility to be achieved between levels of care.

Residential Care

Part 3 of the National Assistance Act of 1948 required Local Authorities to provide residential care for elderly people, hence the term 'Part 3 Accommodation'. Homes can either be run by the Authority themself or by sponsorship in voluntary or privately run homes. Initially, homes were seen to be hotel-type lodgings for fit old people but it is now regarded as preferable to keep this type of person in their own home for as long as possible and residential care on a permanent basis is now normally provided only where a person cannot manage on his own in the community even with domiciliary support and where hospital care is not needed.

In March 1976, about 143,000 elderly people were living in residential accommodation taking into account Local Authority, voluntary and private sectors. Of these, 113,000 were receiving residential care under Part 3 of the National Assistance Act on a permanent basis. Also admitted that year were 37,500 short-stay residents. The present guideline for the number of places available is 25 per 1,000 elderly in the community. The age of new residents is rising and they include more physically and mentally infirm. In the year ending 31 March 1976 nearly 80 per cent of new admissions to Local Authority homes were over 75 and nearly 35 per cent were over 85 years of age. This has brought increased responsibility for the staff and the need for more specialised training.

In general, the type of person admitted to Part 3 accommodation should be reasonably well and mobile. He should be able to use a toilet, attend for meals, dress himself and find his way to his bedroom. Some degree of disability is, however, usually present; for example, the resident may need to use a Zimmer frame or need minor nursing attention. There have always been people with mild degrees of mental impairment in residential homes but care must be taken not to include too many of these, as an unfavourable environment may be created for the more lucid residents. Assessment of an old person for admission to a residential home is therefore important and can cover many aspects.

The real criterion is that the care necessary is not available in the old person's own home and the degree of urgency will have to be critically reviewed on this basis. The idea of a waiting list is probably obsolete and a weekly assessment by social service staff is necessary to balance the various claims of those needing admission. General practitioners can often help in making these decisions by giving accurate and up-to-date medical assessments. Other factors such as the suitability of the home, adequate staffing and geographical location will also have to be taken into account. Co-operation between the various professional workers dealing with the old person and the family is vital in finally determining where an old person is best looked after.

Once an old person enters a Local Authority Home on a permanent basis, this becomes his residence with built-in security of tenure. He can stay there until either he dies or is admitted to hospital. Financial arrangements will vary and will depend on the person's resources and income. This also needs careful discussion before final arrangements are made with both the prospective resident and the family, as often it involves selling his previous home.

Sometimes, but not often, an elderly person who has been resident in Part 3 accommodation achieves a substantial recovery and can once again sustain an independent life in the community. When this happens, because that person is occupying a residential place which is in heavy demand, Local Authority Departments of Social Services and Housing will co-operate to find a fresh home for the person concerned, probably in a sheltered housing unit.

There are a wide variety of buildings used as old people's homes. Some are modern and purpose-built, but others are converted old houses of various sizes and can even date back to the old Poor Law days. It is important that they are attractive and that the old person can identify it as his home. Some authorities allow an old person to bring with him articles of furniture or at least sentimental articles to decorate his room. The management should provide an environment in this way which enables an old person to lead as normal a life as possible. Independence with dignity is vitally necessary for the well-being of an old person and particularly so in an institution. Units where patients undertake their own cooking, laundry etc. have been introduced successfully in many residential homes and this adds to the feeling that an old person can at least do something for himself. All residents should be encouraged to join in outside as well as inside social activities and take part in the running of the home. Such things as looking after their own room and helping in the garden might well be encouraged. How effective this is depends upon the head of the home and the staff. They are expected to provide care which is appropriate to a residential setting and equivalent to that provided by a caring relative. This may well include help with washing, bathing, toileting and care during illness but would not involve long-term nursing care and for this reason it is perhaps better that the head of the home should not be called Matron. Nursing and medical care should be provided by the primary health care team. Some doctors continue to look after their patients in welfare homes but, increasingly, one doctor is prepared to take on the care of all the residents. Privacy and confidentiality should be maintained on medical matters within the home. Other services such as provided by chiropodist, optician or dentist should be made available in the usual way. Many heads of homes are qualified nurses, but this is not necessary as the physical care required by residents is that which would normally be provided by relatives. The real expertise of the staff lies in the field of interpersonal relations. A social work qualification is valuable. For heads of homes an appropriate qualification would be the Certificate of Qualification in Social Work (CQSW) and for residential care staff, the Certificate in Social Services (CSS). This will, however, depend on the function of the establishment and in some homes both may be applicable. The head will usually be recruited through promotion and therefore his or her qualification will be either CQSW or CSS plus management training.

Apart from permanent residence, short-stay accommodation is often available for old people who might have some temporary domestic difficulty. Holiday relief for relatives often falls into this category. Sometimes, too, an old person benefits from a short trial stay at the home. This enables him to test out the idea of permanent residence and makes the sometimes traumatic transition from home to welfare institution easier. Similarly, patients transferred from hospital to a welfare home will need special care and understanding in the first few weeks of adjustment.

Private homes are also available in the community and are often run by voluntary societies. Residents may be supported in these homes by the Local Authority. It is sometimes difficult for these establishments to take severely dependent residents because of lack of suitable staff or premises. In these cases collaboration may be necessary between statutory caring bodies to enable these places to be used more effectively. Joint financing might help if transfer to a home means better utilisation of a hospital bed.

Joint financing can also help in many other ways where co-operation is required by Health Authorities and Local Authorities. It is designed to allow the limited and controlled use of resources available to Health Authorities for the purpose of supporting selected personal social services spending by Local Authorities.

Social Casework

The nature and extent of possible social casework which may be undertaken amongst the elderly can only be briefly touched upon here. It has been said that the social problems experienced by old people are practical rather than emotional, at least on the surface, and it is physical help which is needed rather than supportive casework. However, this is debatable and it is likely that old people experience the full range of emotional problems and help may be needed by them or the family to manage these difficulties.

Sometimes specific groups in a community, as, for instance, old people living in sheltered housing, may need social support to smooth out the interpersonal differences which may occur. An obvious example when people live in a close community is rivalry for friendship or sub-group formation. Sometimes an old person may be excluded from social intercourse for reasons which are at first not clear. These types of problems involve deep analysis and attempts to restore social balance are often very time-consuming. Long-term support may be necessary and this can sometimes be achieved by using group activity, especially at day centres. Rehabilitation of patients discharged from hospital or welfare homes can also be helped by these means.

Social workers can also help to develop the community's awareness of the problems of old people. They can create 'good neighbour' schemes and identify trouble spots where perhaps an area consisting of a high proportion of elderly residents is being persistently vandalised. The aim in these circumstances is to make the community socially self-supporting. The work involves some subtlety and it is important to avoid segregating the elderly from the rest of the community. Integration is the principal objective.

Voluntary Organisations

The Social Services can co-ordinate the activities of voluntary bodies interested in old people, but these organisations also act independently. Most were set up to fulfil a specific need and are often registered charities. Visiting services are provided and group activities such as clubs, good neighbour schemes and outings are arranged. These activities are very valuable in increasing local interest in the welfare of old people. Whilst at the club each person can be assessed for such things as nutritional state, general health and capacity for self-care. Socially isolated people can be helped to acquire new friends and when they do not attend, they can be visited to see if there are problems. Above all, they provide interest and education. Although the addresses of local organisations interested in the welfare of the elderly can be obtained from Area Social Service Departments, help may also be obtained from Age Concern at the following address:

AGE CONCERN,
Bernard Sunley House,
60 Pitcairn Road,
Mitcham, Surrey CR4 3LL.
(Tel: 01-640-5431)

Laundry Services

Most local authorities provide laundry service to assist those caring for old people, particularly if incontinence is a problem. This is usually free. Special incontinence pads and equipment are also available through the Community Nursing Services.

Extra Heating, Extra Diet, Help with Transport Fares

Local Authorities, through their Social Service Departments, may provide additional heating for an old person's house if this is considered necessary. Also, in some parts of the country, help is available with extra diet and in some cases, concessionary fares are available for old people. Finance is usually arranged through the Local Authority.

Adaptations to Houses

These can be arranged by the Social Services Department if they are considered necessary to help the old person. For example, help may be obtained in installing lifts or shower units, and the widening of doors to take a wheelchair.

Aids and Appliances

These are provided by the Social Service Departments and are described in Chapter 11 on Rehabilitation.

Blind Register

Social Service Departments are particularly interested in blind people. The details of the criteria for inclusion on the Blind Register and resulting benefits are described in Chapter 17.

Financial Assistance for the Elderly

A wide range of financial help is available for old people. It is impossible to quote actual levels of benefits as these change frequently to keep up with inflation. Excellent booklets are available from the Local Offices of the DHSS, or from the Information Division, Leaflets Unit, DHSS Block 4, Government Buildings, Honeypot Lane, Staines, Middlesex HA7 1AY. A brief account is given of the benefits of interest to old people, but this is not necessarily meant to be complete. Other information and direct help with specific problems can be obtained from local DHSS offices and in the Age Concern leaflet, 'Your Rights'.

Basic Retirement Pension

Providing that they have satisfied contribution conditions and have retired from regular work, retirement pension is payable to men at 65 years and women at 60 years. At 70 for a man and 65 years for a woman it is payable whether they have retired or not. Retirement pension is paid to a married woman on her husband's contribution when he retires and draws his pension provided that she is over 60 and has retired from regular work other than her domestic duties, or she has reached the age of 65. If a woman qualifies for a pension in her own right as well as her husband's, she receives whichever pension is the higher. From April 1979, under the provisions of the new State Pension Scheme, an additional earnings related pension will be available to those who have not contracted out. By deferring retirement beyond the usual age, extra pension can be earned. Graduated pensions are payable to those who have contributed to the scheme between 6 April 1961 and 5 April 1975. This can also be increased where retirement is deferred. Earnings affect the amount of pension received. Non-contributory retirement pensions may be paid to anyone who is 80 or over, if they are not getting a National Insurance Retirement Pension or equivalent benefit. A pension may be payable to a woman whose husband or former husband was born before 6 July 1883, providing that he is or was entitled to a non-contributory Retirement Pension.

Supplementary Benefit

This is a non-contributory benefit and is payable to people over state pension age. It can supplement state pensions and those from private sources. The entitlement is based on the balance between a person's requirements and resources. The calculation of these is complicated but is well set out in DHSS leaflets. Of interest to the aged are special considerations given to circumstances like the need for special diet, extra heating and domestic help. In calculating capital resources, the value of the old person's house is ignored and also capital below £1,250 and its income.

Widow's Benefit

Widow's benefit takes various forms and is dependent on the husband's contributions record. Widow's allowance is payable for 26 weeks following the husband's death and at the end of that period, no further widow's benefit is payable unless the widow qualifies for widowed mother's allowance, widow's pension or widow's retirement pension.

Widowed mother's allowance is payable to a widow of any age with a child which is accepted as being included in her family.

Attendance Allowance

Attendance Allowance is payable to adults, and children over the age of two who either physically or mentally are severely disabled, the need having been present for at least six months. Medically the person must be so severely disabled that another person is required to give through the day, frequent attention in connection with bodily functions or continual supervision to avoid substantial danger to the disabled person or others; and by night, prolonged or repeated attention, again to bodily functions, or continual supervision to avoid danger. Two rates are payable, depending on whether night or day requirements are satisfied. This allowance is particularly helpful to old people where one or other spouse is severely disabled.

Invalid Care Allowance

Invalid care allowance is paid to people of working age who cannot work because they have to stay at home to care for a severely disabled relative. The benefit is non-contributory, and married women cannot generally qualify for this allowance. Special conditions are applicable to the allowance and there are clear definitions of who constitutes a relative, how many hours a week of caring is required and what is meant by a severely disabled person. This allowance may help an unmarried daughter forced to stay at home to look after an elderly relative.

Rent and Rate Rebate and Rent Allowances

There are various schemes available which provide financial assistance for both owner-occupiers and tenants, including those in Local

Authority dwellings. That is:

(a) owner-occupiers may qualify for rate rebate;
(b) local authority tenants may qualify for rent rebate and rate rebate;
(c) private tenants may qualify for rent allowance (similar to rent rebate) and rate rebate.

All these rebates and allowances are administered by Local Authorities. Whether or not one would qualify to receive any financial benefit from these schemes depends upon a calculation which takes account of the amount of rent and/or rates payable, the level of the household income and financial commitments, plus the size of the family. However, no assistance can be obtained by those in receipt of Supplementary Benefit, which always contains an element in respect of rent and rate commitments for householders, unless it can be seen that someone would be clearly better off by receiving rebates/allowances rather than Supplementary Benefit.

Death Grant

Death grant is a contributory benefit payable to a representative of the deceased. It is normally paid to the executor or administrator of the deceased's estate, or the person who has actually paid or accepted responsibility for the funeral expenses. Payment is limited to the amount of the funeral expenses and any balance is paid to the next of kin.

Free Prescription

Exemption from payment of prescription charges is the entitlement of men over 65 and women over 60. People with Supplementary Benefits are exempt from payment for certain glasses, wigs and fabric supports, dental treatment and dentures.

Hospital Fares for Visitors and Patients

Persons receiving Supplementary Benefit who are attending NHS hospitals can claim refund of their fares when they attend for out-patient treatment, are admitted for in-patient treatment or are discharged after in-patient treatment. In exceptional circumstances, a person who has to visit a close relative in hospital may get help with fares.

Housing the Elderly

Owner-Occupied

A substantial number of old people own their own homes. This is true of most European countries and even more so of the United States. About 47 per cent of elderly persons live in dwellings owned outright by themselves or their spouses, although there are some regional variations. These houses are usually the old family home and have been occupied for some considerable time. Undoubtedly, old people prefer the independence of owning a house and are reluctant to move, even when the residence is becoming obviously unsuitable and financially extending. Situations arise where old houses are badly in need of repair. Under these circumstances Local Authorities can help by making financial grants for necessary work and improvements to be carried out. This is best done on a voluntary basis in agreement with the owner.

Rented Accommodation

From Table 4.4 it can be seen that a sizeable number of old people live in rented accommodation. However, most of those paying rent do so to a Local Authority. The elderly in these houses have usually been in them for a long period of time, although there is usually a larger turnover than in owner-occupied houses as it is easier to persuade old people to move into smaller and more convenient accommodation when there is not the sentimental tie of home ownership. Local Authority housing departments are able to facilitate this type of movement. In recent years, government policy has encouraged Local Authorities to build special housing for old people and an increased number of new houses have been of this type. Additional central government finance has helped this development. This is partly to redress the imbalance caused by the previous concentration on family house production.

Sheltered Accommodation

The provision of sheltered accommodation for old people has also been a development of recent years. The units can be of a bungalow type, but also may be two- or three-storey blocks of flats. An average of about 36 dwellings would constitute a unit together with a warden to supervise. Sometimes there are communal eating and meeting facilities and laundering. Living in these sheltered units can provide certain advantages such as cheap TV licence rates. Many have intercom and alarm bell systems. Units with these latter facilities are best used to meet the needs of less active elderly people. The warden's job is basically that of a good neighbour who will summon the assistance of other services and relatives if necessary. She is not expected to do any nursing or give domestic help, but more to check that individuals are coping and not developing illnesses or being neglected.

On occasions, sheltered housing units have been built near a Part 3 residential home, thus enabling the tenants to receive the benefit of support and attention from the highly qualified staff of the residential home, and yet maintain a more satisfying state of independence. If increasing age brings about a general deterioration, then the move into the residential home can be far less traumatic than is often the case.

Housing Associations

Housing associations or trusts were first established in the early part of this century as charitable bodies, to cater for those with special housing needs, including the elderly. Larger national associations such as the Anchor Housing Association and the Hanover Housing Association cater specially for the housing needs of the elderly. There are variations in the type of accommodation provided, some schemes involving groups of flats or, as in the case of the Anchor Association, the objective being to provide warden-supported sheltered housing. Some societies, such as Abbeyfield, aim to provide the elderly with their own rooms within the security and companionship of small households. All are registered charities and non-profit-making bodies. Legislation exists to promote and regulate the housing association movement.

There are one or two pilot schemes nationally, supported by government, to allow the elderly to use capital receipts from sale of homes, to buy long leases of sheltered flats. They then pay rent but it is not too high and the usual rebates/allowances apply. They may have some cash over to provide some comforts. At a time of economic constraint this type of scheme has potential and is likely to become more widespread.

Information

Information for this section of the book has been derived from DHSS Leaflet FBI, November 1977, *Family Benefits and Pensions.* It is recommended for further reading. A *Complete Catalogue* of Social Security leaflets is also published (Leaflet N1 146, November 1977).

Further Reading

Arrangements for Old Age, Consumers' Association, 14 Buckingham Street, London WC2 6DS (1972).

Residential Homes for the Elderly. Arrangements for Health Care (Department of Health and Social Security Welsh Office, 1978).

Meals for the Elderly, The King's Fund, 14 Palace Court, London W2 4HT (1978).

C.P. Brearley, *Residential Work with the Elderly* (London, Routledge and Kegan Paul, 1977).

Eric Butterworth and Robert Holman, *Social Welfare in Modern Britain*, 3rd impression (London, Fontana/Collins, 1978).

Muriel Brown, *Introduction to Social Administration in Britain*, 4th edition (London, Hutchinson, 1977).

Age Concern, *Your Rights*, 5th edition (1978).

Age Concern (Greater London), *Housing Advice for the Elderly* (1978).

10 NURSING THE ELDERLY IN THE COMMUNITY

At the present time a nurse can work in the community in two ways. First, she can be employed by a general practitioner as part of his ancillary staff and work within the practice premises. A nurse working in this way is known as the practice sister. Second, she can be employed by the Area Health Authority as a community nurse or community nursing sister and work on the district in people's homes. She was previously known in this context as the district nurse. Community nurses are usually attached to several general practices and they form a team of a community nursing sister, always an SRN, and two SEN nurses. There may also be other auxiliary nurse helpers to carry out tasks such as bathing a patient. All are members of the primary health care team.

Modern medicine is absolutely dependent on nursing help both in hospital and in the community. When dealing with a sick old person, it is essential to involve the community nursing sister at as early a stage as possible in the illness so that as well as providing care and therapy, she can also prevent certain problems and complications from developing. Special difficulties are presented by nursing old people at home. They are often frail and suffer from multiple pathology. There may be mental impairment present, so that instructions may not be fully understood. A task that could quite easily be carried out by a younger patient may be beyond the ability of one more elderly. Drugs may be forgotten and tablet-taking may be quite haphazard and irregular. Old people may be lonely and cease caring for themselves. Nurses may be the only visitors to motivate them and to attend to diet and hygiene.

In the community, nurses are called on to care for three types of case. First, there is the acutely ill old person with, for instance, bronchitis. This needs the full range of general nursing care but usually only for a limited time. The aim in this type of case is to restore him to full health and his normal place in the community. Secondly, the nursing services may be involved in the long-term maintenance of, for instance, a patient who has had a stroke. Here, the sufferer may be ambulant but nevertheless require some nursing care to supervise such things as contractures of healing pressure sores. Thirdly, there is the nursing of the chronically ill or bedfast patient at home. A whole variety of cases may be involved, ranging from discharged surgical patients, especially those with genito-urinary problems, to the terminally ill. Maintenance of elderly diabetics may be necessary and also the routine dressing of leg ulcers.

Basic Principles of Nursing a Patient at Home

As has been mentioned, it is essential for the nurse to arrive early on the scene. Nurses should educate their doctors to alert them at the beginning of an illness, and not leave it until it is obvious to all that nursing care is imperative. The room where the patient is to be nursed needs to be adequately heated and lighted. It is sometimes more convenient to nurse an ill old person downstairs than in a cramped bedroom. This may also be easier for the family and facilitates earlier rehabilitation. At home the bed is often too low – but can be raised with blocks. It must be at a height which is safe for the patient to get in and out of. Ideally, when he sits on the edge, his feet should be flat on the floor. Occasionally, safety sides are necessary when there is danger of the patient falling out of bed. It is possible to obtain hospital beds with sides for use in the home, and these should be installed if possible, as makeshift arrangements are seldom satisfactory. A bed table is also helpful, especially a cantilever type with adjustable height and angle. Bedding needs to be light and warm. Some people prefer duvets but they can be difficult to keep clean. Sheepskins are available and many find them very comfortable. Old people slip down the bed easily and at home ingenious relatives have sometimes been able to fix overhead handles for the patient to clasp. A rope ladder attached to the end of the bed can also be helpful in some situations. In general old people should be encouraged to stay in bed for as little time as possible. This minimising of bed rest is a fundamental precept in nursing old people. As the patient recovers, the relatives will need instructing as to how best to get the patient in and out of bed. There are special gadgets such as hoists available for moving very disabled patients at home, although hospital admission may be necessary when this is very difficult. Usually a patient can be helped to swing his legs over the side of the bed until he is sitting upright. After a pause, he should be able to stand. The patient will also need help with dressing and undressing at this stage.

Dehydration can occur all too easily in elderly people and adequate fluid intake is necessary. The diet also needs supervising with special care to ensure that sufficient vitamins are taken. Toileting arrangements are important and the nurse may well have to resort to certain aids such as the use of a commode, so that toileting is easy and comfortable. General attention to personal care such as washing, bathing, shaving and hairbrushing is necessary. This helps the patient to preserve his self-respect. It is important that an old person be treated as an individual; for instance, if possible, bed-bathing should be kept to a minimum and he should be encouraged to wash himself and allowed to use his own bath or shower. Clothes too, should be kept clean and changed frequently.

Community nurses have a very special responsibility in supervising treatment. Tablets need to be taken regularly and a watch kept for side-effects. This is much more difficult at home than in hospital, where there is the traditional drug round and total nursing supervision for the whole 24 hours of the day. At home, this is impracticable and the nurse has to rely on members of the family or neighbours to undertake general supervision. This involves her in the task of educating these helpers in what needs to be done and what signs of change to watch for. If these extra helpers are not available when a patient lives alone, night sitting and home help services may be possible; but if not, it is sometimes better for the patient to be admitted to hospital.

In the community the nurse might find herself very much concerned with other tasks apart from straightforward nursing. She may well be asked to undertake simple physiotherapy, including training a patient to use aids. Occupational and speech therapy may also be necessary, particularly for those suffering from stroke. This general rehabilitation role of the community sister is very important and can be the critical factor which successfully leads the patient through acute illness back to independence.

Very often an old person's perception of the environment is retained even when bedfast, and recovery may be helped by bright and cheerful surroundings as well as the general encouragement of those giving nursing care. Some may become very dependent on the nurse and this applies even more so in the community than in hospital. A dilemma sometimes exists as to how firm one ought to be in insisting that certain tasks should be undertaken by patients themselves and how much to do for them because of their disability. It is sometimes very easy to do more than necessary in order to save time. The hospital geriatric team can often help if this is a problem.

The Social Services Departments will provide aids and appliances to make nursing in the home easier. These include chemical toilets, commodes, tripods, Zimmer frames, monkey chains to make moving up the bed easier, high chairs, bath seats, hand rails and ramps. The

Community Nursing Service will provide equipment for the comfort of patients in bed, including disposable sheets and pads. Kanga pants and pads for those suffering from incontinence are also provided. In general, the Social Services Departments provide aids to living and the nursing services provide aids to nursing, but there is some overlap. The Marie Curie Foundation makes allowances to patients suffering from cancer for extra diet and other comforts and is also very helpful in providing night sitters.

Records

Communication is helped by nursing records being left at the patient's home. Temperature charts are unnecessary but notes made of temperature and pulse in acutely ill patients are useful. The doctor should also record changes in treatment. Messages can be left on the record sheets. However, there is no real substitute for direct verbal communication between doctor and nurse.

The Community Nurse and the Clinic for the Elderly

If a clinic for the elderly is in existence, the community nursing team should be involved in its work. Any home nursing requirements should be accepted and the community sister should be available for discussion about ongoing nursing problems. Liaison with the geriatric community nurses attached to the hospital department can also be achieved through such a clinic so that a smooth handover of responsibility can be effected when a patient is finally discharged back into the community. Acute situations can be discussed with the doctor and other helpers. It is only usually necessary for the nurse to be present for about half an hour at the point when case discussions and reviews are being held, so that a great deal of her valuable time is not absorbed.

Geriatric Community Nursing Team

Geriatric hospital/community nursing liaison teams are available in some areas. They visit patients in their own home after discharge from hospital, offering support and advice, particularly to relatives. Their duties are fundamentally to liaise with hospital, medical, nursing and social staff and their counterparts in the community. They also make special visits to those on the waiting list for admission to hospital. Supervision of continuing rehabilitation of discharged hospital patients may also be part of their duties.

The Practice Sister

The practice sister usually works from the surgery and ideally has a treatment room at her disposal so that she can treat ambulatory old people. The range of care might include the giving of injections, dressing ulcers and dealing with injuries. General supervision of treatment may also be undertaken, for instance for patients with hypertension or diabetes. Again, an old person may be referred from the clinic for the elderly for specific treatment such as ear syringing or for treating eye infections.

Special Nursing Problems

1. Pressure Sores

Pressure sores can be either superficial or deep. Superficial sores are usually due to small injuries of the skin and can be caused by moving a patient up the bed; they are usually painful. They are the most common form of ulcer and may account for up to 90 per cent of the total. They may become infected and this is particularly liable to occur where urinary incontinence is also present. Deep sores, which are sometimes called decubitas ulcers, are much more serious and occur when the skin over a bony prominence is compressed for any length of time. This causes the blood supply to be cut off with resulting tissue destruction. This may occur without the skin surface actually being broken, and discolouration may not immediately appear. Nevertheless, extensive damage may have occurred to the underlying tissues. They are said to be painless, but this can be very variable and often they can be painful, especially over the heel. Areas particularly vulnerable to developing this type of sore are over the main bony prominences such as the upper part of the femur, the buttocks and the lower part of the back. They can occur over the shoulder blades and elbow. The resultant sore is usually deep and can sometimes be covered by a hard scab which hides the necrotic changes which have taken place underneath. Other factors also contribute to the development of ulcers. Incontinence can cause skin sogginess. Unconscious and paralysed patients are vulnerable as well as those who are thin and emaciated. Arteriosclerosis can reduce the blood supply to the skin and make infarction more likely. Fever, dehydration and poor nutrition may also be contributory. The use of a hot water bottle may sometimes cause a burn which may become infected and ulcerated.

Prevention of Sores. Bed sores, both superficial and deep, are in many ways a tragic occurrence and as they are so difficult to treat, prevention is of prime importance when nursing old people. Damage can often be done in the first week of the illness, or even overnight, and therefore prevention should be instituted early. The period of bed rest should be reduced to a minimum and the position of an old person changed as frequently as possible. This may have to be as often as every two hours in an unconscious paralysed patient. There may of course be a danger of developing a pressure sore on the buttock if the patient is got out of bed too soon and made to sit in a chair without being able to move. Special care should also be taken to keep the skin clean and it is beneficial to apply a little light massage. Soap and water is undoubtedly better than the traditional rubbing on of methylated spirits and powder applications. Barrier creams such as Vasogen (Pharmax) and Conotrane (WBP) may be used to protect vulnerable areas. This can also be achieved conveniently by using an aerosol spray of which Sprilon (Pharmax) is a popular example, especially when there is early reddening, although it is expensive to use continually. The general condition of the patient obviously needs attention with a special watch kept for dehydration. A diet rich in protein and with added vitamins is helpful. If incontinence is a problem, an indwelling catheter may become necessary. Sedation should be avoided so that the patient is capable of moving naturally. Any pressure should be relieved and attention should also be paid to the skin areas which are vulnerable, especially for early changes in colour. Heel sores can develop when the patient finds it difficult to move his legs because of tight sheets, and a cradle may prevent this.

Many special beds have been developed to help in the prevention of sores and are considerably more sophisticated than the original sheepskins. Few, however, are of much value in the home. Ripple or alternating pressure mattresses can be used, but although perhaps saving the nurses' time they do need careful supervision and a reliable electricity supply. New technical developments are producing beds which may eventually solve the problem, ranging from hammock types to a continuously inflated air mattress. They are expensive and it will possibly be a long time before they are seen in the patient's home.

Treatment. Superficial sores should be cleaned with soap and water or a non-irritant lotion such as Cetrimide 1% and after being allowed to dry, sprayed with Sprilon. Healing usually takes place slowly, although sometimes infection may be present and then a swab should be taken for bacteriological assessment. However, antibiotics are not usually necessary.

Deep sores need to be cleaned and necrotic tissue removed. This can usually be done using a forceps and scissors but powders are available such as Debrisan (Pharmax) to soften the slough. Sometimes it is helpful to dissolve the powder in a little glycerine. Debrison is expensive and cheaper products include Aserbine (Bencard) and Malatex (Norton). Simple Eusol cleaning is, however, often effective. Surgical treatment is rarely needed in old age, but if the ulcer is extensive and the patient's condition good, surgical advice about the possibility of grafting may be justified.

2. Urinary Incontinence

Causes. Incontinence may be due to diseases of the brain or spinal cord (neurogenic) or local abnormalities in the bladder and urinary tract (focal). These produce different types of bladder abnormality. Cases of neurogenic urinary incontinence characteristically have a hypersensitive bladder which empties frequently without the patient being aware of this taking place. The bladder is not usually palpable as its capacity is reduced and it is small and contracted. On the other hand, focal lesions which interfere with the emptying are usually associated with a full bladder and overflow incontinence. The patient wets himself but on examination a full bladder is found. Causes can include such things as urethral caruncle, urinary infection and prolapse in the female, and prostatic hypertrophy in the male. Constipation may be a cause of both. Associated with these are overlying emotional and environmental problems. It sometimes happens that a patient in an acute period of stress may be incontinent but once this is passed full continence returns. Some environmental changes such as going to hospital or sleeping in a strange bed can precipitate incontinence, often with great embarrassment to the old person. Severe illness of any sort can produce incontinence, particularly if the patient is becoming terminal. Diabetes mellitus may be an associated finding. Because of increased frequency and reduced bladder capacity in old age, immobility is a potent background cause of incontinence. This may, for instance, occur after an operation.

Treatment in the first place involves dealing with any local lesion and help from a urological or gynaecological surgeon may be necessary. Rectal examination may reveal faecal impaction which is causing the condition. Chronic constipation may also need to be treated. Infections, if present, should be remedied, and bacteriological examination of the urine is necessary, either by obtaining a midstream specimen, or if this is impossible, by catheterisation. Glycosuria should also be excluded. Full urological examination may be necessary, including intravenous pyelography and cystoscopy.

It may prove impossible to control the incontinence by treatment and this is when management becomes important. There is little joy in dealing with an incontinent old patient and it may be tempting to show distaste and annoyance at the continual unclean and wet state. Some old people even give the impression they are incontinent on purpose as an attention-seeking device. This is rarely the case and much can be achieved by understanding the problem and urging the patient to keep as active as possible. In the first place, therefore, the patients should be treated sympathetically and with general reassurance, remembering that they are often extremely embarrassed by their problem. Steps should be taken to make sure that the bladder is emptied at regular intervals. This may be difficult, particularly when half-hourly bladder emptying is necessary and it is frustrating when immediately after a visit to the toilet, the patient again, involuntarily, passes urine. It is helpful to make sure that the patient has adequate recourse to perhaps a bedside commode or bottle, particularly at night. Sedatives are best kept to a minimum and restriction of fluid in the evening may be valuable to patients suffering from nocturnal incontinence.

There are a number of drugs used in the treatment of incontinence. Anticholinergic drugs (Atropine-like) permit increased relaxation of the bladder and an increase in volume. Ferguson Anderson suggests Propantheline bromide (Probanthine) 30 mg four times a day and Emepromium bromide (Cetaprin) 100 mg three times a day. The side-effects are retention of urine, blurring of vision and dryness of mouth. He also suggests the use of an incontinence chart so that the pattern of micturition can be anticipated and the drugs prescribed accordingly; it is also useful to monitor progress. The dosage may need to be changed or the combination adjusted. If there is no progress, the treatment would have to be discontinued. When depression is present incontinence may be helped by antidepressant drugs, for instance Amitriptyline (Triptizol) 25-50 mg at night.

Despite these measures the condition is often persistent and recourse has to be made to incontinence aids. Disposable incontinence pads are very useful for the patient in bed and they can absorb up to 300 ml of urine. The person should sit directly on them without intervening clothes. For this reason they are not suitable for use when patients are sitting in a chair. Disposable napkins or pants are available and a variety very popular with patients are Kanga pants. They ingeniously hold the pad in a waterproof pouch outside the pants which are made of a one way water repellent fabric which allows the urine through into the disposable pad. About 400 ml of urine can be held and there is no need to remove the pants to change the pad. Some local authorities arrange for the disposable pads to be collected from the house at intervals. In the male, penile clamps or condom drainage is sometimes helpful. Special care of the skin is always needed in these cases. Permanent catheterisation is sometimes necessary. The plastic balloon catheter is the one usually used. The balloon is usually filled with sterile water, using a 20 ml syringe. Infection is always the risk with this type of catheter and even with an inflated balloon, patients can sometimes pull it out. Noxyflex Solution (Geistlich) should be instilled into the bladder if infection is present, either weekly or on alternate days. Long-term antibiotic therapy is not used routinely with elderly patients. Foley's balloon catheter needs changing monthly but the new Silastic or Dover's catheters need only to be changed every three months and are a great improvement. Although always a difficult task, nursing this type of patient at home is now much more feasible because of the new improved catheters.

3. Faecal Incontinence

This is a distressing condition which often occurs in bedfast demented patients. It is commonly due to faecal impaction and produces spurious diarrhoea. Neoplasm of the bowel is another possible cause. Short-term incontinence may be associated with an attack of diarrhoea caused by infection of the bowel or dietary disturbance. Any serious illness may be associated with faecal incontinence and some drugs such as antibiotics and iron may cause diarrhoea in an old person and precipitate incontinence. Self-prescribed large doses of laxatives are not uncommon in the elderly and may produce diarrhoea. Nursing treatment involves attention to any predisposing causes and relief of the impaction if present. This usually involves enemas or rectal washout and sometimes manual removal. Suppositories, for instance either Dulcolax (Bisacodyl) or glycerine, may be helpful, as also are the Microlax enemas (SKF). Laxatives such as Dorbanex (Riker) or Normacol (Norgine) may be used, but liquid paraffin is best avoided. Many patients rely on Senokot (Reckitt and Colman) tablets or granules. It may be helpful to increase the volume of the faeces by using a high-residue diet containing bran. Certain foods cause diarrhoea in some patients and if these can be recognised, they should be avoided. If diarrhoea is persistent once infection or neoplasm have been excluded, Kaolin mixture may help to harden the stools. General attention to training and suitable clothing should be instituted as outlined in the section on urinary incontinence.

4. Avoiding Contractures

When nursing a bedfast or partially bedfast old person, it is important to realise how easily contractures may develop. A stroke patient may be discharged back home and without careful supervision may very quickly develop a contracture. They are usually associated with prolonged stay in bed and when this is inevitable, active and passive movements of the limbs which are at risk should be encouraged. If the joints are painful, analgesics should be given to allow them to move more freely. Bedclothes should not be pulled tightly around the legs as restriction of movement can sometimes cause knee-stiffening or foot-drop.

5. Nursing a Restless Patient

There are many causes of restlessness in an old person. Infections, particularly pneumonia, or any acute illness, and also such conditions as heart failure and anaemia may make an old person sleepless. Impairment of consciousness often associated with brain failure and developing cerebral thrombosis can aggravate the condition. Uraemic patients may be particularly fretful and disorientated at night. Certain drugs used in sedation may give rise to agitation and this is particularly true of bromides and barbiturates. Other drugs may also be responsible and therapy should be reviewed when restlessness is present. Pain and discomfort may contribute and may result from a full bladder or faecal impaction. Old persons who will not settle at night are well known to nurses. They may be reasonably co-operative through the day, but once the evening arrives, they may noisily wander around, upsetting everyone by their disorientation. Tranquillisers are helpful and the most usual ones used are Sparine and Largactil, both in syrup form. General measures, such as keeping the patient up during the day and ensuring some activity, not going to bed too soon, and providing a bedtime milky drink may, however, be all that is necessary.

Conclusion

Nursing the elderly at home is therefore a task which demands the full resources of nursing skill. There are special difficulties involved and this demands understanding on the part of the community nursing team to achieve success. Apart from nursing, the tasks undertaken by the community team involve rehabilitation, patient education, attention to diet, and keeping an eye on the general social state of the patient. There are also special problems which have been outlined which make nursing old people a challenge.

Finally, the nursing team should of course be an integrated part of the primary health care team, and work closely with its other members.

Notes and Recommended Further Reading

1. 'Treating pressure sores', *British Medical Journal*, vol.1 (1978), p.1232.
2. W. Ferguson Anderson, *Practical Management of the Elderly* (Oxford and Edinburgh, Blackwell Scientific Publications, 1971).
3. Dorothy Mandelstam, *Incontinence: a Guide to the Understanding and Management of a Very Common Complaint* (London, Heinemann Medical Books, 1977).
4. R.E. Irvine, M.K. Bagnall and B.J. Smith, *The Older Patient. A Textbook of Geriatrics*, 3rd edition (London, Hodder and Stoughton, 1978). This is a textbook mainly for nurses and describes well the principles of nursing care in hospital for old people, but has little about domiciliary nursing care. Nevertheless, the nursing procedures are well described and much relates to home nursing.
5. Bob Browne, *Management for Continence* (Liverpool, Age Concern, 1978).
6. Charlotte R. Kratz, *The Care of the Long-term Sick in the Community* (Edinburgh and London, Churchill Livingstone, 1978).
7. Alison F.M. Storrs, *Geriatric Nursing* (London, Bailliere Tindall, 1976),

11 REHABILITATION AND RESETTLEMENT

Rehabilitation of sick old people has probably been one of the most neglected areas in the care of the elderly in the community. The reasons for this are diverse, but have included a shortage of the necessary paramedical workers and an absence of co-operation between these workers and both nurses and doctors. The situation, however, is improving. More rehabilitation resources are becoming available in the community, often as an extension of the hospital services, and there is a growing realisation of their importance amongst doctors and other members of the primary health care team. Early discharge from hospital and the increased number of cases being treated at home is also stimulating the demand for domiciliary rehabilitation services.

The aim is to convert the patient from a state of dependence because of illness to one of independence with the ability to live a normal existence. This is sometimes impossible but, nevertheless, considerable benefit can be gained by effective rehabilitation. Medical treatment of illness is naturally very important, but side by side with this must go the task of restoring functional ability. This may involve learning or relearning basic skills.

In the community, there are two types of situation demanding rehabilitation. One is when patients have been discharged from hospital and where procedures to restore function have been started but need to be continued in the home. It is sometimes tragic to see the effects of the hard and dedicated work done in the hospital which has enabled the person to return home being rapidly reversed by failure to maintain and continue the process once he is back in the community. There is what might be termed the hospital/home continuum and the transition from one to the other needs careful supervision. The co-operation of both hospital and community services is essential if this resettlement is to be successful.

The second situation is where the person is treated at home in the first place and where rehabilitation is needed to enable him once more to lead a normal life. In the elderly this is particularly important because even minor illness can reduce the capacity for self-care and unless this is realised full recovery may never take place. Illnesses such as stroke may lead to major disablement and demand considerable rehabilitation, but conditions such as heart failure, pneumonia, bronchitis and urinary tract infection, where the patient may be confined to bed for some time, also run risks of the patient developing muscular weakness, joint stiffening and general loss of mobility and hence need similar attention.

Assessment

It is important at the very onset of an illness to get some idea of what the future holds for a particular patient. The consequences of an illness in terms of loss of ability to self-care must be remembered and assessment of the physical, mental, psychological and socio-environmental condition of the patient must be made with primarily functional ability in mind. It is useful in this respect if the person's previous state and circumstances are known.

Physical assessment involves general examination to determine functional capacity, especially looking at such things as muscular power, grip and mobility. Attention must also be given to cardio-respiratory function, vision and hearing, as these may well have an effect on what a patient can do. A stroke will often mean the possibility of only limited mobility or an inability to perform activities in the home. Heart failure ma may cause breathlessness, and this again will prevent performance of certain heavier tasks. Special situations may exist which may demand extra management by the patient, and he will probably need teaching about these. For instance, incontinence may be present, or there may be the necessity to look after a colostomy. There may also be a requirement for a special diet, and this needs to be taken into account during the assessment of how someone is likely to cope. A speech defect may make it necessary to assess the patient's power to communicate. His ability to read and write will need testing, as well as the capacity to interpret sign language.

Whether a patient can look after himself both now and in the future also needs to be determined. Can he feed, wash and bath? Can he dress and undress and attend to his general grooming? Will he need help with toileting? How will he manage at night? Will he be able to walk safely and unaided? Can he prepare meals for himself and could he do the housework and shopping if necessary? Will he be able to launder his clothes?

The patient's mental state also needs determining. Intellectual impairment following a stroke or concomitant senile dementia may also reduce functional ability. Depression or anxiety state may be present, and many old people react to illness by losing self-confidence and respond with despair to the thought of losing independence. A fairly active old person may be reduced to being a housefast prisoner for these psychological reasons. It is also important to discover changes in perception of body image as deterioration in this can affect functional performance.

A careful look needs to be taken at the patient's home environment. The type of house he lives in may determine how he is to cope. Will it suit his new needs? If not, can it be adapted? The attitude of family and neighbours is also important. Some relatives are unwilling to accept the burden of looking after a disabled old person and it might be that such antagonism will reduce the chance of effective rehabilitation. Admission to a welfare home may sometimes be necessary for these reasons.

These are the type of questions which will need to be asked in order to plan physical rehabilitation and factors need identifying which might interfere with this. Realism is essential when assessing the prospects of an old person, and only obtainable goals should be pursued. Many tasks are physically possible but the patient may be unable to cope because of poor understanding, failing vision or lack of motivation. Cooking, for instance, may be dangerous. Rehabilitation services therefore must aim to achieve only what is feasibly consistent with the patient's abilities. To this end, assessment should be an ongoing exercise and the team should critically monitor progress and be aware of changes in the general condition of the patient. Old people go in and out of illness and what can be done today may not be possible tomorrow.

The Team

Rehabilitation involves many people working together as a team. This should ideally consist of a doctor, a nurse, a physiotherapist, an occupational therapist, a speech therapist and a medical social worker – each with equally important contributions to make. Help may also be given by a dietician, a chiropodist and a hairdresser. This latter is often a very helpful morale-booster and may make a vital contribution to improving the patient's outlook. Relatives, neighbours, voluntary workers and clergy can also be integral members of the team. The patient himself is of course a crucial member and should be consulted at all stages and informed about the ideas behind the various procedures. In hospital, the help of most of the professional workers is available, although, depending on the illness, all may not always be required. Speech and communication problems, for example, may not be present. At home, there may only be the doctor and community nurse available but, if possible, other expert help should be brought in at an early stage.

The family and the patient can often co-operate with the team and understand what is happening during rehabilitation and should contribute to the early assessment. Some simple rehabilitation techniques are described later, and may be useful when resources are limited.

Each member of the team should be interested in the general condition of the patient and in the progress he is making, but each also has a distinctive contribution to make. The *doctor* of course has the responsibility for medical treatment, but also must act as co-ordinator of the many other activities. In hospital, it is usually the consultant in charge who undertakes these tasks, and in the community, it is the general practitioner. Close co-operation between these two is essential, especially at the time of resettlement into the community. The GP should know what is going on and be in a position to continue with rehabilitation at home. The previous relationships between him and the patient can often be very important in re-establishing confidence and giving the patient the willpower to succeed in adapting to home life after hospital discharge. Where someone has been treated at home, the general practitioner must arrange and co-ordinate the services, and supervise rehabilitation himself.

Nurses, either in hospital or at home, are vital in providing a person with the confidence necessary for restoring normal living, as well as looking after his nursing needs. At home, they may be the only ones available for undertaking these tasks.

Physiotherapists and *remedial gymnasts* usually work in a hospital rehabilitation unit, but are sometimes available to treat a patient at home. When this is the case, there is the advantage of their being able to evaluate needs in a real-life environment. The physiotherapist's main concern is with mobility and here she has first of all to gain the patient's co-operation. She must aim to prevent and correct muscle deformity and wasting. Also normal muscle usage must be strengthened and loss of balance improved. The idea is to reduce incoordination and enable the patient to walk unaided.

Occupational therapists are also essential to recovery and are concerned with enabling the patient to cope with such tasks as dressing, undressing, eating, drinking, shaving, cooking, cleaning, toileting and personal grooming. They have suffered in the past from being thought to be merely teachers of handicrafts which might relieve the patient's boredom.

Occupational therapy naturally follows on from physiotherapy but should really occur simultaneously. Teaching the patient finer movements and skilled activities can start when the patient is learning to become mobile again. The patient's co-operation once more is necessary, and it should be explained to him that it is part of the programme to restore him to full activity. Occupational therapy is excellent for the patient's morale and gives him a sense of achievement when something has been successfully undertaken.

Speech therapists are concerned with communication and the problem is often a difficult one. All possible methods should be used to help and can include reading, writing and sign language. The sense of touch as well as sight should also be exploited. Speech problems are very frustrating to a patient. A paralysed limb may be endurable, but failure to relate to another person can be intolerable. Restoring this capacity is very important and very much the work of the speech therapist. It is unfortunate that these professionals are in relatively short supply. The Chest, Heart and Stroke Association Stroke Clubs are, however, useful venues for continuing speech therapy.

Social workers and medical social workers are concerned with the social and environmental background of the patient. When he is being looked after at home, it is the community social worker who is responsible, but in hospital there is usually an attached medical social worker. She becomes of crucial importance in easing the patient from hospital back into the community and usually follows him up for a short period. Co-ordination of the various stages in this and gaining the help of other paramedical workers is the task of the medical social worker and her encouragement is often supremely important to both patient and relatives.

A whole range of social problems may need to be solved whether a patient is nursed at home, or is being transferred from hospital. Housing may be unsuitable and full of hazards and there may need to be adaptations. Various aids and appliances such as Zimmer frames may need to be provided. Communications may be difficult and a telephone may need to be installed. Financial problems can exist and there may be difficulties with diet and heating. Patients may have unsatisfactory relationships with family or neighbours, and houses may have been vandalised during the hospital stay.

Many services may need to be arranged by the social worker, for instance, the provision of meals on wheels and home helps. It is sometimes beneficial for a patient who is convalescing, to have a holiday or a day trip out, and these can often be arranged in co-operation with voluntary bodies. Workshops and social community centres may also be helpful in the final stages of rehabilitation. Sometimes, supportive casework is necessary for families and this may be needed particularly when there are psychological stresses present.

These then are the members of the basic rehabilitation team and it is important that all should co-operate and communicate. Workers in hospitals should have good liaison with workers in the community. Supervised home visits for patients in hospital before they are discharged and trial weekends are very useful in resettling a patient back into the community, and are also good for achieving co-operation. Members of the hospital team are in a sense becoming part of the domiciliary team in this way and it is a development which needs to be encouraged.

Simple Rehabilitation in the Home

Sometimes the family alone, perhaps with the help of the community nurse, is faced with undertaking the patient's rehabilitation. These circumstances, which usually involve a patient suffering from a stroke, should be restricted to mild cases only. The rehabilitation process should start as early as possible in the illness and will usually begin when the patient is in bed. Simple passive exercises for the affected limb should be undertaken with the aim particularly of avoiding contractures. Gentle massage will help the patient to feel more comfortable and may give the affected muscles extra tone. Unaffected limbs and muscles must also be exercised to prevent disuse atrophy. Special care must be taken of the shoulder of a hemiplegic stroke sufferer. It can very easily be deranged by relatives or other helpers when lifting the patient with either the hand in the axilla or holding the paralysed arm.

Speech therapy, where necessary, can also begin at this stage and the patient can be encouraged to articulate words. It may be possible to arrange for him to start reading or at least listening to the radio. As part of early occupational therapy, such things as knitting or jigsaw puzzle-solving may be introduced. As soon as practicable, the patient should be encouraged to sit in a chair. This is feasible when he is able to sit without falling. Special attention should be given to the chair and it should have a seat with a surface parallel to the ground. The seat should be about 18 in.(46 cm) from the floor. A firm back capable of support is necessary and it is essential for it to have arms. The chair must of course be stable. At home it is probably better that it should not have castors and trays are best avoided. The front legs should not have a connecting bar as this prevents the old person putting his feet back when rising.

Once the patient is capable of sitting in the chair, passive movements should be continued and he can start to learn how to dress as an extension of his occupational therapy. Movements of the hands and fingers should be encouraged and he can sit on the edge of the bed or chair and move his feet up and down. The next stage is standing and this is sometimes difficult if balance is impaired. If this is so, expert physiotherapist help is usually required but sometimes the relatives, giving ample support, can teach him how to stand and then proceed to help him to walk. The use of walking aids such as a Zimmer frame or tripod are often useful in helping old people to gain confidence. Gradually and with encouragement, the patient should be able to achieve this mobility and at the end be able to manage for himself the tasks of general care. Where there are more complicated problems of contractures, or movement is severely restricted, expert help should be obtained and, if necessary, admission into a hospital rehabilitation unit arranged.

Aids and Appliances

The patient may need various aids and appliances to help him to regain independence, and if full recovery is impossible, these may become permanent features of his life. Rehabilitation involves assessing which aids will be needed, and also teaching people how to use them. Aids are usually small, easily handled items and if the device is larger and non-portable, it is usually described as a piece of equipment. The word 'appliance' is used to describe an aid which is purposely made for the individual.

The idea of these aids is to enable a person to do something which would otherwise be difficult or impossible. Their function is to enable him to overcome the effects of a disability and be more independent. The aids themselves must be of the best design possible and they should be efficient. They should be cheap but this does not mean shoddy or unattractive. Robust equipment is important, because anything which is likely to break will quickly lose the confidence of the user. Too many aids should be avoided as the confusion brought about by too much technology can be a danger.

The number of aids devised is endless. Many are home-made and involve considerable ingenuity. Some useful aids are described under each basic care heading.

Toileting. To be able to use the toilet is important to a patient's self-respect. If the toilet is too low, this can be raised with a plastic seat. Rails can be placed on either side to help with sitting and standing. If it is impossible for a person to use a pedestal toilet, a commode, bed-pan or bottle may be necessary.

Washing. Washing the upper part of the body is usually no great problem but reaching the back and feet may be difficult and long-handled brushes and sponges can help. Getting in and out of the bath may be quite impossible, but some old people can manage with bath rails and a bath seat. Non-slip mats are essential in a bathroom. A shower is often useful.

Shaving and Grooming. Shaving can be a problem for an old man and an electric razor with a long handle may help. For women, application of make-up may be helped by a long-handled lipstick holder. Similarly, combs and brushes can also be attached to long handles.

Dressing. It is obvious that disabled old persons should wear suitable clothes, avoiding buttons, preferably using zips and having everything fastening at the front. Tights and trousers for women are easier to put on, having the added advantage of extra protection and warmth and they may also hide artificial limbs or calipers. Shoes should be of the non-lace type. Various aids are also available for picking up items from the floor and also for putting on stockings.

Feeding. When feeding is a problem because of poor grip or lack of co-ordination of hand movements, cutlery with large handles may help; drinking may be facilitated through a straw or in a special cup which cannot be knocked over. Plates with stable wide bases may make things easier and there are many devices for dealing with jugs and teapots. Non-slip table mats are also useful.

Mobility. Many aids are available to help with mobility. For support there are simple walking sticks, Zimmer frames, tripods and quadrupods. Wheelchairs are available either through the Social Services Department or directly through a GP, using form No.AOF 5G. Walking can also be assisted by shoe raises, surgical shoes and calipers with toe-raising springs or inside irons and T-straps. Modifications to the house are sometimes possible and these can include support rails, levelling out of steps and providing ramps and widening of doors. Hoists are also occasionally provided to help old people out of bed and into a wheelchair. The British Council for the Rehabilitaton of the Disabled has established an organisation known as Rehabilitation Engineering

Movement Advisory Panels (REMAP). Specific problems of individual mobility can be helped by these voluntary panels which are planned to function nation-wide.

Household Duties. There are many specially adapted cooking utensils. Split level cookers are helpful, and electrical sockets should be at appropriate heights. A device may be attached to taps to make them easier to turn on. Long-handled brushes and dusters can aid cleaning as also can vacuum cleaners.

Communication. There is a range of devices to help communication. If a person is unable to speak clearly, a pencil and pad should be nearby. There are aids to help with writing, including, if appropriate, a typewriter. Reading can be helped by bookrests and books with large type. A telephone may be necessary and if this is needed to summon medical help urgently, the Social Services Department may finance this. The Post Office can also advise on special telephones for the disabled and details can be found in the telephone directory. Alarm systems or even whistles may be installed to enable old people to attract attention if necessary.

Hobbies. Many disabled old people like to continue with their hobbies. Help may be available from voluntary organisations. Gardening, for instance, may be possible using specially adapted tools.

Maintenance after Rehabilitation

Having successfully rehabilitated an old person after an illness, especially if aids have been introduced to assist in this, it is absolutely essential to maintain some supervision. There is a considerable risk of deterioration if the stimulus of a professional worker is withdrawn too quickly. The work of several months can be lost in several weeks if the patient becomes apathetic. Some form of general supervision is therefore vital, so that any difficulties can be spotted early and the cause found and corrected.

Further Information

Further information on aids can be obtained from:

The Disabled Living Foundation,
346 Kensington High Street,
London W14 8NS.

British Gas gives information about gas aids for the disabled. Electricity Council gives information about electrical aids. The Chest, Heart and Stroke Association is also able to give valuable assistance.

Further Reading

Graham Mulley, *Stroke – a Handbook for the Patient's Family* (Chest, Heart and Stroke Association, 1978).

Stephen Mattingley, *Rehabilitation Today* (London, Update Publications, 1978).

Sydney Foot, Handicapped at Home (Design Centre Book, published in association with the Disabled Foundation, 1977). This book gives excellent information about useful organisations and further reading.

Margaret Johnstone, *The Stroke Patient. Principles of Rehabilitation* (London, Churchill Livingstone, 1976).

Margaret Hawker, *Return to Mobility* (Chest, Heart and Stroke Association, 1978).

Susan Hooker, *Caring for Elderly People: Understanding and Practical Help* (London, Routledge and Kegan Paul, 1976).

12 DRUG TREATMENT FOR THE ELDERLY

Most doctors are aware of the tendency to prescribe large numbers of drugs for elderly patients and they are also aware of the demand from some old people for drugs to alleviate their multiple symptomatology. As has already been mentioned, multiple pathology is the rule in old age and old people, despite unreported need, once faced with the doctor, expect him to prescribe for all of their many complaints. The pressure on the doctor to give drugs can be quite considerable. At the same time, most doctors, nurses and social workers have had the experience of finding an old person at home with a large number of bottles of tablets on the mantlepiece, only to discover when moving into the kitchen or bathroom an equally large number of bottles on shelves and in cabinets. The old person is all too often unaware of what the tablets are for; many of them have been in his possession for a long time and his taking of them is frequently quite irrational and haphazard. This is not only confined to patients at home. When visiting welfare homes or private nursing homes, it is remarkable to see the long lists pinned up in the office of drugs which each old person is taking or supposed to be taking. There is thus a situation where large quantities and types of medicines are prescribed for old people, and perhaps the time has come to review the whole policy of drug therapy for the elderly. Ivan Illich, in his criticism of the medical profession, points out that one out of every five patients admitted to a typical research hospital acquires iatrogenic disease, often as a complication of drug therapy.[1] How much similar disease is being caused in the community by careless prescribing is unknown.

Physiological and Pharmacological Background

In old age, changes occur in certain physiological functions which can affect the action of drugs in the body. Absorption normally takes place from the gastro-intestinal tract and ageing may reduce the blood flow to these areas and the number of absorbing cells. There is no direct evidence, however, that absorption is seriously reduced in old age. Metabolism normally occurs in the liver, where drugs are broken down to inactive forms prior to excretion via the kidney. Some drugs are excreted unchanged. In old age, both the liver and kidney can become less efficient in undertaking these processes, and this can lead to slower elimination of drugs from the body and they can therefore remain active for longer periods. This natural physiological ageing process can be augmented by disease. Renal and hepatic illness can reduce drug elimination, as can general conditions such as heart failure or dehydration. Reduction in overall body size associated with old age may affect the distribution of drugs in the body. Tissues may alter in their response to certain drugs, a good example being barbiturates, where sedative effect on the brain may be increased. Old people therefore can be expected to be more sensitive to the effect of drugs and suffer more often from side-effects. Drug interactions of a synergistic or antagonistic nature may also be increased.

Dangers of Drug Therapy in Old Age

It is hard to determine in an individual patient whether physiological changes will have occurred sufficiently to cause increased liability of side-effects or incorrect dosage. Actual chronological age may outstrip biological age and an old person may retain perfectly efficient physiological mechanisms. Nevertheless, the danger must be appreciated and watch kept for possible over-treatment. Not all drugs are affected by these changes. In general, preparations used as replacement therapy need to be given in normal doses and, indeed, there is sometimes the danger of under-treatment. For instance, in thyroid deficiency, it might be that too low a dose of thyroxine is being given to achieve the ideal therapeutic effect. Without being aware of these problems, the doctor is at risk of wrongly prescribing for his old patients, and this can be made more difficult by a person's own habit of self-prescribing. Sometimes large numbers of proprietary preparations are taken alongside the doctor's medicines. There is even a chance that old people are given drugs by friends and relatives which were originally prescribed for (and have done good to) other people.

There is also the problem of whether old people take their prescribed treatment properly. Some do not understand the tablet-taking regime and, as a high proportion of old people are responsible for their own medicine-taking, it is hardly surprising that many do not take their treatment as intended by the doctor. This is particularly true of patients living alone who are not receiving any regular supervision.

Under these circumstances, problems with adverse drug reactions are not uncommon. This has been highlighted by Professor James Williamson, who carried out an investigation for the British Geriatrics Society into hospital admissions at 42 geriatric departments.[2] Of the admissions, 2.8 per cent were necessitated solely by the adverse effects of drugs and 12.4 per cent of the patients had adverse reactions of some kind. It appears that all doctors are faced with the problem, as Professor Williamson found that the level of adverse reactions amongst the patients being referred to geriatric wards from other departments in the hospital was the same as in patients being admitted from their homes.

General Principles of Drug Therapy in Old Age

It is of prime importance to make an accurate diagnosis. Only with this will effective treatment be possible. Difficulties arise, however, in old people, because of the presence of several illnesses and these can often interact with each other. Some diseases are not amenable to treatment and some are perhaps better left alone. The doctor should have realistic aims when treating old people, and the effect of the drug given must be clear and have a purpose. This often means drawing up a system of priorities so that perhaps only the most important conditions and those most likely to respond are treated. A minimal number of drugs should be used and if larger quantities are necessary, they should be given only for as short a time as possible. Other treatments apart from pharmacological ones are sometimes possible. Occasionally, changes in diet, attention to social difficulties and simple physiotherapy can be just as effective as drug treatment. The effect of arranging twice-weekly visits to a luncheon centre can dramatically improve the outlook (and often the appetite) of a lonely old man. Oedema can disappear once mobility is restored. Above all, the reassuring presence of the doctor himself is often therapeutic.

The pharmacological action of the drugs used should be known to the doctor. He should be aware also of the correct doses for an old person and the possible side-effects and interactions of the drugs he is using. It is useful to have regard to the body-weight of the patient and adjust the dose accordingly as in the case of children. The use of placebos and the purely symptomatic treatment of illness is sometimes necessary but this should be kept to a minimum and preferably used only for a limited period. Drugs which are likely to be beneficial should not be withheld just because a patient is old, but sometimes it is obvious that the effect of the drug on the patient is worse than the sumptoms being treated, and it is better to cease treatment in these circumstances. In fact, it is sometimes more important and beneficial to take patients off treatment than to start new courses of tablets.

Alleviation of the Problem

Many problems would be alleviated by adherence to the general principles of prescribing outlined above, but there are also organisational difficulties, an obvious one being the practice of repeat prescriptions. An old person on a drug needs reviewing at moderately frequent intervals. Side-effects may arise which the patient himself will not report. Shaw and Opit, studying the medication of 127 randomly selected patients aged over 70, found that about half the patients were on long-term treatment.[3] Nineteen had no recorded contact with the family doctor for six months or longer, and examination by nurse surveillance suggested that three might be suffering from drug toxicity. They concluded that reliance on self-referral by elderly patients was unsafe. Periodic review of elderly patients on long-term treatment is therefore essential.

Drug compliance in the elderly can also be improved by education. Many devices have been recommended for improving patient understanding of their medication. Instructions can be written down or transferred on to a calendar. A tablet identification card is helpful to augment written instructions. Supervisors can give the patient his daily supply in a small box and check can be made later to see if they have been taken. Special packaging can be used with tablets marked for each day. Pharmacists can be helpful in giving specific and clear instructions to old patients and the habit of hoarding tablets could be reduced if the date of dispensing was noted on the label. A difficulty arises sometimes when patients are given tablets which have an unfamiliar appearance because they have been produced by a different drug manufacturer. The patient thinks he has been given a different drug and treats it with some suspicion and this is particularly true of patients discharged from hospital. The treatment of these patients needs to be carefully reviewed by the doctor and a check made that the patient is taking the tablets as instructed. The problem of approved names and proprietary names is also difficult for an old person to understand. Co-operation cards, showing the current treatment and always available on the patient, are useful in co-ordinating advice and therapy. The patient should be asked directly about any other medicines or pills which he is taking. Simplicity of treatment is essential; if one tablet can take the place of three, so much the better.

Some Specific Drugs

For a full account of use of drugs and their side-effects, textbooks of pharmacology and geriatric medicine will need to be consulted. A brief review is given here of some of the problems associated with commonly used drugs. Discussion of the drugs used in the treatment of diabetes, hypertension, rheumatic conditions, Parkinson's disease and relief of severe pain are discussed in other chapters.

Digoxin

Digoxin has always been a useful drug in the treatment of heart failure, although these days duretics have become the first-line therapy for the condition, especially in old age. Digoxin is excreted slowly and tends to accumulate. Adverse effects are therefore possible, and the dose needs to be continually monitored. The blood level of Digoxin can now be estimated and should be at about 1.5 μg/ml. The drug should only be used as long as the clinical indication remains and usually old people do not need to be kept on Digoxin for too long. Frequently, Digoxin is used together with oral diuretics and these may increase its toxicity. This is even more likely if there is potassium deficiency and blood levels should be monitored in patients receiving Digoxin and diuretics. As the dose of Digoxin needed by the elderly is low, the 0.0625 mg (paediatric) tablet is useful.

Diuretics

Diuretics are frequently prescribed for old people, although not all oedema responds to this therapy. They are also used to treat hypertension, but this should only be done with care, because of the risks of sudden hypotension, although this is minimal with diuretics. The dangers of acute retention and incontinence also increase with age and the speed of action of the drug. Most of the commonly used diuretics require potassium supplements, particularly when Digoxin is also being used or the diet is likely to be low in potassium. Latent diabetes may be precipitated by diuretic therapy and the risk increases with age. The development of gout is also a possibility. When there is difficulty in taking potassium tablets, as when a patient is unlikely to co-operate reliably, a potassium conserving preparation should be used and a good combination is Amiloride hydrochloride 5 mg, in combination with Hydrochlorothiazide 50 mg (Moduretic). It may however cause high blood potassium levels. Commonly used diuretics are:

Bendrofluazide 2.5 mg or 5 mg (Aprinox)
Frusemide 40 mg (Lasix)
Chlorothiazide 500 mg (Saluric).

Vaso-dilators

These are used in old people to counteract the effect of arteriosclerotic disease, both in the brain and the peripheral circulation. Whether they are effective is open to question, but patients often improve symptomatically and the group of drugs seems to be without serious side-effects.

Commonly used vasodilators are:

Thymoxamine hydrochloride 40 mg (Opilon)
Cyclandelate 400 mg (Cyclospasmol)
Inositol nocitanate 500 mg (Hexopal)

Hypnotics

Barbiturates are poorly tolerated in old age and apart from treatment of epilepsy, they should not normally be used. They sometimes cause confusion and unsteadiness. Restlessness at night can occur and this may persist for some time after the drug is withdrawn. When changing to another type of sedative it is best to do this gradually by slowly reducing the dose of barbiturate. If sedation is required, the initial dose should be small because of the risk of sensitivity.

Commonly used preparations are:

Nitrazepam 5 mg (Mogadon)
Chlormethiazole (Heminevrin) 500 mg
Dichloralphenazone 650 mg (Welldorm)

Tranquillisers/Antidepressants

The most widely used tranquillisers are diazepam (Valium) and chlordiazepoxide (Librium) but in more severe cases chlorpromazine (Largactil) and promazine (Sparine) are often preferred. Largactil may cause liver damage. More potent drugs are best avoided in elderly patients unless given under psychiatric supervision. The dose needs to be small initially and maintenance judged according to response. Depression is common in old age and antidepressants can be useful. Tricyclic antidepressants are widely used, and may be given in a single dose at night. They have some sedative effect and therefore can help the old patient to sleep. There is a wide variety of possible interactions between tricyclic and other drugs and it is wise to review other treatment before prescribing. Tetracyclics with fewer side effects, are now recognised as an improvement on tricyclics.

Patients should also be warned about avoiding alcohol and the necessity to inform the dentist of any treatment they are taking, particularly if anaesthesia is contemplated. Tricyclic antidepressants have atropine-like side-effects and may cause constipation.

Commonly used anti-depressants are:

Amitriptyline hydrochloride 25 mg (Tryptizol)
Imipramine hydrochloride 25 mg (Tofranil)
Dopthiepin 25 mg (Prothiaden)

Conclusion

The pharmacology of modern drugs is, in general, extremely complex and is particularly so in old people. This chapter has in no way attempted to detail the many pssible side-effects of drugs used. The range is wide, as are the possible interactions. Doctors should know about the problems of the drugs they find useful. Good accounts are given in a modern textbook of geriatrics or of pharmacology.

Notes

1. Ivan Illich, *Medical Nemesis. The Exploration of Health* (London, Calder and Boyars, 1975).
2. James Williamson, Paper to British Geriatrics Society, 1977.
3. S.M. Shaw and L.J. Opit, 'Need for Supervision in the Elderly Receiving Long-term Prescribed Medication', *British Medical Journal*, vol.1 (1976), pp.505-7.

Further Reading

J.C. Brocklehurst, *Textbook of Geriatric Medicine and Gerontology* (London, Churchill Livingstone, 1973).
T.G. Judge and F.I. Caird, *Drug Treatment of the Elderly Patient* (Tunbridge Wells, Pitman Medical, 1978).

PART FIVE: SOME COMMON SITUATIONS

So far, the care of the elderly has been discussed in general terms, but this section will look at some specific examples of illnesses which occur commonly in old age. They have been chosen for this reason and also because they are examples of conditions which need both acute care and often long-term maintenance and follow-up. They are therefore illnesses which are very likely to be seen at a clinic for the elderly.

It is not the intention of this section to be a complete textbook of conditions found in old age. Indeed, many of the minor illnesses found at clinics are not included. It is also not a list of possible unreported diseases; some, such as heart failure, are not mentioned. However, mental illness, problems with mobility and special senses are commonly allowed to go by default amongst old people.

A theme underlying the choice of subjects has been the opportunities given to describe preventive action and also the possibilities of demonstrating the team role in management, either acutely or in maintenance and rehabilitation. Both these aspects are clearly present, for instance in the chapters on mental illness and stroke. Hypothermia and nutritional problems are included because of the chances of discussing them at clinics for the elderly.

The clinical details given are based on experience gained in working amongst the elderly in general practice and may not be identical with those described in textbooks of medicine or geriatrics. Nevertheless, it is hoped that they give a fair account of the conditions as they are seen in the community.

13 MENTAL ILLNESS IN OLD AGE

Mental illness in old age has attracted very little interest from doctors and a good deal of superstitious misunderstanding from the general public. The result is that it has come to be regarded as a subject as difficult as any in the whole of medicine. Why should this be? Probably the underlying reason is the fact that a mentally ill old person presents, often inconveniently, as a particularly difficult type of patient, with background problems which are seemingly insoluble and which can be expected to deteriorate. Management is often arduous and time-consuming. Given this, it is not surprising that many doctors are not interested in treating mentally sick old people, particularly when the rewards of a successful outcome seem to be minimal. Yet a mentally disturbed old person poses a serious problem which demands considerable knowledge and skill to manage. Perhaps some satisfaction can be gained from using these to bring a measure of relief to the patient and also to the family.

Diagnosis of mental disease in old age is sometimes difficult and there are often physical and social components to the illness. Many cases are unreported to general practitioners until late in the course of development and there are reasons for this. First, the insidious nature of the development of some forms of mental illness and the fact that mental deterioration may be accepted as part of old age makes relatives slow to realise that help is required. Secondly, groups of old people such as those living alone are particularly vulnerable to some forms of mental ill health (for example, anxiety state and paraphrenia) and tend not to report the problem because the infirmity itself takes away the initiative required. Thirdly, the relatives are often embarrassed by the thought of mental illness in the family, with all the stigma of lunatic asylums, and hence they are reluctant to seek advice.

Prevalence

Mental illness of all types is common in old age, but the exact prevalence is not clear. Early surveys showed that about 10 per cent of old people in the over-65 age group were demented and in the over-80 age group this proportion was as high as 20 per cent.[1] Tom Arie has estimated that the average general practitioner's list is likely to contain between 30 and 40 demented old patients.[2] There is also a high prevalence of other forms of mental illness, particularly depression and acute anxiety state. Even if the number arising in each age group each year remains the same, the sum total of mentally sick old people is likely to increase because of the overall population growth.

Acute Crisis Situations

By far the largest practical problem confronting community health and social workers is what has come to be called an acute psycho-geriatric crisis. This unfortunate label implies a very dramatic event, but this may not necessarily be so. Nevertheless, it is true that mental illness in old age often presents in a sudden and unmanageable way. The story told at the beginning of Chapter 5 could well have applied to a mentally ill old person. The mental condition is usually described as one of confusion and may be an acute episode in a chronic dementia, or might be an acute delirium. Terminology is difficult in this area and in particular there are problems with the word confusion. It is probably best regarded as a descriptive word and not as a diagnosis. Someone may be 'confused' when they manifest disorientation of place and time, or, in other words, when there is cognitive impairment. The term 'confusional state' is sometimes used as the name of a syndrome but it is really synonymous with the condition known as 'delirium'.

Causes of Crisis

1. Background Causes. These are factors which contribute to the development of a crisis but are not the illness itself. They are usually concerned with the provision of basic care to the patient and occur when this care is unavailable or withdrawn. Inadequacy of services may also precipitate an acute situation and this has sometimes been called a 'GP frustration' crisis. The doctor dealing with the situation finds himself getting little help from either the hospital or Social Services but is faced with continual representations from relatives, neighbours, shopkeepers and even town councillors to 'do something about' the old person. A great deal of strain results and the doctor is tempted to manipulate a crisis so that help can be obtained in a more dramatic, but perhaps not absolutely necessary form; and this usually means an attempt to seek hospital admission. Sometimes this is in effect treatment for the doctor's problem. An example of this was the case of an old lady who regularly rang late each evening confessing some serious crime which she had committed earlier that day. She usually contacted the police as well, but was hurriedly told to get in touch with her doctor! In this type of category also comes what Tom Arie calls the preventive crisis which may also be referred to as the 'Friday afternoon crisis'.[3] Here the doctor sees a potentially difficult problem late on a Friday and being anxious to have it resolved seeks urgent hospital admission. This may be a form of preventive activity and perhaps hospitals should recognise this; but equally, the doctor should be quite willing to accept the patient back into his care once the initial problems have been sorted out.

2. Precipitating Mental Causes. Although any mental condition can produce crisis, the most common precipitating mental illness is acute delirium. This is a clinical state characterised by confusion. There is usually physical restlessness, disordered comprehension of the environment and disorientation in time. Relatives may be unrecognised by the patient.

Causes of Acute Delirium

1. Toxic. These can include acute infection, toxaemia (as for instance caused by toxins absorbed from a gangrenous limb) and alcohol.

2. Cerebral Conditions. Stroke can present as delirium with or without other signs of cerebral damage. Dysphasia, if present, can add greatly to the patient's problems. Any condition which reduces the oxygen supply to the brain such as heart failure, anaemia or chronic lung disease may produce confusion. Certain vitamin deficiencies may contribute to the condition. Increased intra-cranial pressure from causes such as tumour may also be responsible but usually there is a longer period of developing personality change.

3. Endocrine Conditions. Thyroid deficiency occasionally presents as the so-called myxoedematous madness. This condition was originally described by Richard Asher and made famous by A.J. Cronin in his novel *The Citadel*. Complications of diabetes are not uncommon in old people and both hypoglycaemia and hyperglycaemia can cause delirium, and the risk may be greater when oral hypoglycaemic tablets are used.

4. Drugs. The altered response to drugs in old age makes them an important cause of delirium.

5. Social Stress. Apart from social stresses on the family in provision of care, social problems experienced by old patients themselves can also precipitate an episode of acute delirium. Worry about finance, health or housing are good examples. Psychological stress caused by family disputes, or problems with other members of the household can affect an old person and produce breakdown and delirium. Sometimes harassment due to vandalism or threatening behaviour by teenagers can also have the same result. Sometimes even physical attack can result in subsequent psychological trauma, leading to delirium.

Management of Crises

Assessment and Diagnosis

It is of prime importance to make a diagnosis of the patient's condition. A very careful history needs to be taken and here a GP is in a very privileged position. Knowledge of the background of previous illnesses, treatment currently being taken and the possibility of family stress is invaluable. The time course of the condition also needs to be known. Unfortunately, sometimes the GP is unaware of these for reasons described earlier. The overall condition of the patient needs assessing, including noting physical illness and making an appreciation of the social and environmental circumstances. A careful look needs to be taken for underlying background and precipitating causes.

Action

Often acute crises may be managed effectively at home by the community health team, particularly with the help of a social worker. Occasionally, however, expert psychiatric or geriatric help is required. Ideally, this should take the form of a case conference at the patient's home, where, as well as the specialist, the nursing and social worker members of the team should be present. Unfortunately time often does not allow this to happen.

It is necessary first to identify needs, and the resources that are available to satisfy them. Provisions for care and the feasibility of undertaking treatment and investigation need to be known. Care will usually involve decisions as to whether the relatives and the Social Services can provide basic facilities. Medically, it means assessing whether the GP and nursing service can cope with the necessary treatment. The temptation to admit to hospital may be very strong, but the patient may be harmed rather than helped by this, because of the risks of further confusion due to the strange environment and the development of complications such as incontinence. Short-term admission often turns out to be long-term admission and even if a quick and good recovery is made, the home may in effect have disappeared because of deterioration in the fabric of the house or the fact that previous helpers are reluctant to accept back the old person into their care.

So, if possible, it is better to avoid removal of a patient to the frightening and unfamiliar environment of a hospital, and it is preferable to keep him in surroundings which are familiar and where at least he has a certain amount of orientation. Family and medical resources for looking after him must, however, be sufficient and if there is any doubt about this, admission to hospital is probably unavoidable.

If it is decided to cope at home, attention to any underlying cause of the crisis is necessary and treatment of physical illness must be undertaken. In acute delirium, drugs should be used sparingly, as they can make the condition worse. In a restless patient sedation may be used, but the dosage should be small and a careful watch kept for reactions. The dose needs to be altered according to the response. Useful preparations are chloral hydrate, nitrazepam, chlorpromazine, and thioridazine (Melleril). These preparations have the advantage that they can be given in liquid form. Observation should be made of fluid intake to avoid dehydration. The nursing services should be fully integrated into the management of the case and it is important, particularly where there might have been neglect in the intake of food, to supervise diet and where necessary to give vitamin supplements. Social Services must provide support for the relatives both by supplying practical help and by social counselling.

Particular problems arise where the patient lives by himself and sometimes hospital admission is necessary for this reason alone. But occasionally, when the mental problem is severe or the patient refuses to co-operate, serious difficulties of care result. Certification is sometimes necessary in the latter circumstance. An example might be an old man with mild senile dementia associated with financial irresponsibility. A recent case in the author's practice involved such a patient roaming around with hundreds of pound notes in his pockets. Indeed, his entire life savings were scattered about his person. He was extremely uncooperative but help was obtained from the community psychiatric social worker who took charge of the money and by frequent visiting and gentle persuasion managed to get the old patient to attend a day centre. Difficulties could, however, have arisen.

Finally, long-term supervision is usually necessary once the initial crisis period has passed. Established nursing and social worker services need to be reassessed and placed on a maintenance basis. Voluntary workers can sometimes be enlisted to help at this stage and a day centre may also be arranged. Though not common in the UK, boarding-out of mentally sick old people to foster homes is used in some countries to provide longer-term care. Accommodation may need assessment and occasionally it is best to rehouse the patient or make adaptations to the existing home. If this is impossible, and the person lives alone, admission to a welfare home, particularly one specialising in the care of people with mental disorder, may be the only possibility.

The advice of the specialist should still be available and, in this sense, he should be a member of the team caring for the old person at home. An open mind needs to be kept on the options and it might be that at some future date, because of a rapidly changing clinical situation or failure to respond to treatment, hospital treatment may be necessary. As indicated, day hospital care may sometimes be helpful and has the advantage of avoiding the difficulties associated with admission. Relief for relatives is often considerable when this can be arranged and there is the added advantage of professionals being able to watch patients' response to treatment more closely.

There is now developing (in some districts) an excellent hospital service known as a Crisis Intervention Team. Rather on the lines of an obstetric flying squad, a consultant psychiatrist, a health visitor and a mental nursing officer are prepared to turn out at any time of day or night, as well as at weekends, to give help with an acute psycho-geriatric crisis. Co-operation and assistance from the Social Service Department are usually forthcoming. Expert help on the spot can be very useful for the GP, and often it makes it possible to manage the situation at home by defusing a difficult situation and providing emergency care at just the right time.

Prevention

The preventative aspects of the community health care team's work should include an aim to recognise, at an early stage, mental illness and intellectual impairment. This can be done by running screening clinics for the elderly (described in an earlier chapter) and also by having an alert attitude towards old people presenting for treatment. The importance of knowing what to look for at an early stage of development and the range of possibilities in old people cannot be overstressed. There are also certain 'at risk' groups which are likely to develop mental illness and they need special surveillance. They include people living alone, the recently bereaved and those with social problems, particularly of finance and housing. Patients recently discharged from hospital or welfare homes may well find difficulty in adapting to life in the community and sometimes relapse and develop mental symptoms. The general practitioner is in a special position to be able to recognise the early deterioration of a person's mental condition because of his knowledge of the previous personality. Despite this, it is possible that crises will still occur, but with preventative action, their frequency should be reduced.

Common Clinical Conditions

The broad divisions of mental illness found in old age are given in Table 13.1. The distinctions are not always clear-cut and several conditions may be present simultaneously in the same patient. For example, someone suffering from senile dementia may also be depressed. It is not intended here to give a comprehensive account of each illness, but rather an impression of each so that an idea may be gained as to the range of mental illness in old age. For treatment, textbooks of psychiatry must be consulted.

Table 13.1: Classification of Mental Illness in Old Age

1. Mental Illness	
Organic — confusion	a. Acute delirium
	b. Chronic dementia
Functional	a. Manic depression
	b. Paraphrenia
	c. Anxiety state
2. Personality and Behaviour Disorder	

(after Brice Pitt)

Senile Dementia

This is a condition which results eventually in a complete disruption of the personality. In the early stage, there are minor degrees of intellectual difficulty with forgetfulness a prominent feature. There is a gradual reduction in the ability to learn new skills and adapt to changing environments. The emotions may be disorganised and inappropriate, especially crying or laughing. There is memory loss for recent events but happenings which occurred many years previously may be remembered with what appears to be astonishing accuracy. Objective tests show that these also are impaired, but not so much as new learning, and therefore old learning appears relatively intact. Two types of dementia have been described. One, more common in men, may follow a series of strokes, and runs a fairly definite downhill course with intellectual functions declining in a series of steps. Another type, probably true senile dementia, is more common in women over 75 years and is usually more slowly progressive. The patient's physical condition is often surprisingly good, but when this begins to fail, acute delirium may be the final outcome. This may initiate quite dramatic episodes and is responsible for such situations as where an old person is found wandering around, usually only partially clothed, in the early hours of the morning.

Affective Disorders

These are common in old age and account for up to half the admissions to mental hospitals in the over-65 age group. They consist of the manic depressive illnesses and are associated with a disfunction of the patient's emotional state. Deterioration of intellect may, of course, also be present. The individual presents with a weary air of overall depression and there is often an associated degree of apathy. He may be fearful for his own health and show hypochondriacal symptoms. Worry may also exist about the health of his relatives and perhaps even more so about his own financial and housing difficulties. There may be physical components to the illness and there may be complaints of such problems as lack of sleep, poor appetite and headache. A small percentage, perhaps between 5 and 10 per cent of these patients, exhibit the manic phase of the illness. These people are hyper-excitable, often agitated and highly talkative, going to great lengths to describe the importance of their achievements. Outrageous activities may be embarked upon such as spending a large quantity of money on items like a new car or quite unnecessary pieces of furniture. Suicide is a real danger in a depressed old person, the incidence being higher than in the younger age groups. They feel a sense of unworthiness and no longer want to live: they talk about 'doing away with themselves' and this is particularly likely to happen when they have recently lost a spouse or other relative. They often say they would be better off if they could join the lost loved one.

Paraphrenia

Sometimes patients present in old age with symptoms which are predominantly paranoid, i.e. a feeling of being persecuted in one way or another. This condition was first clearly described by Martin Roth in

1955 and typically develops in old age. Professor Ferguson Anderson describes the patient as 'classically a woman, often unmarried, and frequently affected by disorders of either vision or hearing'. Indeed deafness is said to be very potent in producing the symptoms. The patients who might have had paranoid traits throughout life develop delusions in old age, particularly about neighbours, whom they see as a threat. Others develop fantasy ideas about sex and imagine that they are being watched whilst undressing and even have worries about being molested.

Acute Anxiety State

This is also common in old age. The patients present with the usual worried and agitated demeanour. Bodily symptoms are common and the patient often complains of sweating, faintness, rapid pulse-rate and headache. Indeed, the physical symptoms may predominate. There are usually predisposing causes such as financial and housing worries. Harassment may be a problem and old people, particularly those living alone, may be easily upset by the uncalled-for activity of certain neighbours. A particularly unpleasant case took place recently (summer 1978) when a 93-year-old woman was raped by three young men. Fear of this type of assault can easily induce an acute anxiety state.

Behaviour Disorders and Personality Changes

It has been said that personality defects that are present in earlier life are exaggerated as one grows older and this can be seen quite commonly in the community. A person who has been a little on the ungenerous side becomes, as he grows older, positively mean and miserly. Similarly, one who has been occasionally short-tempered can become extremely awkward and unpleasant in old age. A person who was constantly quarrelling with her neighbours can take this to gross extremes as the years advance. Enemies created in earlier life can take on a more important and sinister aspect and this may apply to relatives. Sometimes there have been hidden jealousies between members of the same family and these come to the surface in old age. These personality changes lead to the patient becoming more inward-looking; the circle of friendships diminishes, and in the end the old person lives a hermit's life and can be quite unapproachable and difficult to help.

There is described amongst in-patients a condition of institutional neurosis where they show apathy and loss of initiative. This is said to be one reason for keeping people out of hospital. It can, however, also happen at home, and the neurosis can equally well occur when a patient is institutionalised in the confines of his own house.

Although old people very rarely consult with sexual problems, the family may come to the doctor with stories of aberrant sexual behaviour. An elderly man may suddenly develop a preoccupation with sex and this may produce difficulties with female relatives or helpers. Sometimes indecent exposure is a problem and occasionally overt sexual advances may be made to any member of the opposite sex who happens to be present. Occasionally, these sexual abnormalities take the form of indecent assault on children. A sexual problem may also manifest itself in quite unrealistic jealousies and can result in physical violence.

Alcoholism is occasionally seen in old age for the first time, and there may be associated features of anxiety or depression. It is necessary when dealing with an acute episode of confusion to bear in mind the possibility of this problem and look for the tell-tale evidence of large numbers of bottles scattered around the house or in the dustbins.

Obsessive neurosis may also develop in old people and they can become completely dominated by such things as cleanliness and the position of various pieces of furniture around the house. The timing of meals will have to be exact, as perhaps will the amount of sleep taken. Sometimes, such obsessions concern physical health and the patient may become absolutely fixed on the idea that he has got a cancer somewhere and frequent visits are paid to the doctor with a whole variety of symptoms. Many X-rays and consultant opinions are called for and the patient, within a few months, can pass rapidly from the ENT Department to the Chest Clinic, to the abdominal surgeon and finally to a neurologist. Very little seems to be able to convince these people that they are, in fact, physically well.

Legal Problems

Incapacity in old people does bring legal problems. When the infirmity is physical and there is difficulty, for instance, in writing a cheque, it is helpful if some relative or some professional person is given Power of Attorney. The purpose of this is to enable some other person (the Donee) to sign documents in the name of the person who has given the power (the Donor). These documents used to be lengthy but are now much simpler thanks to the Power of Attorney Act of 1971. The Authority given to the Donee is wide, but it can be limited to a particular purpose. Once the power has been executed, it can be produced to interested persons and the signature of the Donee will then be accepted in place of that of the Donor.

The Power of Attorney should, however, only be used where the Donor is of full mental capacity and if the old person's mental state deteriorates the existing power will become invalid.

If the elderly person is mentally incapable of managing his own affairs, the proper course is not to use a Power of Attorney but to go to the Court of Protection for an Order. The Court of Protection Office is at Store Street, London, WC1E 7BP, and letters to the Chief Clerk will produce guidance for the relatives of those in this situation. In effect, once the case has been properly investigated and the incapacity of the elderly person established by written evidence from the appropriate medical practitioner, all the affairs of the elderly person are placed under supervision of the Court of Protection and property cannot be disposed of, nor can income or assets be dealt with in any way, unless the Court of Protection agrees. The Court will usually appoint some person known as a Receiver who is often a close relative or, in default, a friend or professional adviser to deal, under its instruction, with the elderly person's property. All transactions in the financial affairs of the person concerned must be dealt with in this way. To avoid frequent applications to the Court, normally an order is made for weekly payments for the benefit of the elderly person, but any disposal of assets such as a house or investments will need the specific sanction of the Court of Protection. The legal costs of obtaining such an Order and of administering it are normally dealt with out of the estate of the person concerned.

Notes

1. D.W.K. Kay, P. Beamish and Martin Roth, 'Old Age and Mental Disorders in Newcastle on Tyne', *British Journal of Psychiatry*, vol.110 (1964), pp.146-58.
2. Tom Arie, 'Dementia in the Elderly. Diagnosis and Assessment', *British Medical Journal*, vol.4 (1973), pp.540-3.
3. Ibid.

Further Reading

Brice Pitt, *Psychogeriatrics: Introduction to the Psychiatry of Old Age* (London, Churchill Livingstone, 1974).

J.A. Whitehead, *Psychiatric Disorders in Old Age* (Aylesbury, Harvey, Miller and Medcalfe, 1974).

J.A. Whitehead, *In the Service of Old Age* (Aylesbury, Harvey, Miller and Medcalfe, 1977).

14 MOBILITY AND FALLS

Loss of mobility can be partial or complete. The prevalence of totally bedfast old people is not high, but increases with advancing age. Relative immobility, which often means the person is housefast, is a common cause of reduced effective health.

Assessment of Mobility

Functional ability is all-important and before examination of the limbs and joints, it is necessary to find out what the old person can actually do. Can he walk unaided, or does he need a frame, tripod or support from furniture? Can he get out of bed, or a chair? Can he stoop to pick things up from the floor? Inquiry must also be made as to how well he can undertake basic personal and domestic tasks. It is also useful to know whether he is able to use public transport, do his own shopping and enjoy hobbies and social contacts.

If diminished mobility has been established by functional assessment, possible causes should be sought by examination. Pain, stiffness and swelling of the joints, and weakness, wasting, rigidity or tremor of the limbs, if present, are obvious and the patient's stance may also be awkward and unsteady. Movements may lack co-ordination. A weak grip may interfere with efficient use of walking aids. Examination of the feet sometimes reveals gnarled toe-nails and twisted joints, which hinder walking and the wearing of properly fitting shoes.

Causes of Immobility

Immobility is always a feature of a disorder; by itself it does not constitute a diagnosis. Pain and weakness are the main reasons for difficulty in movement with perhaps mental apathy contributing to the overall inertia. Pain, which must never be accepted as normal in old age, may arise from bones, muscles or joints. Diseases of these structures producing this effect will be described later. Weakness arises from a wide number of possible causes. Neurological disease can produce actual muscle wasting and lack of co-ordination. Two examples of this are motor-neurone disease and Parkinson's disease. Disorders of the heart and lung also contribute to immobility by causing breathlessness, ankle-swelling, chest pain, or pain in the legs on walking. General debility may result from endocrine, renal and blood diseases and reduce a patient's ability to move around. The patient's mental state, if impaired, also contributes to inertia, and visual and hearing difficulties can have the same effect. Over-sedation and the side-effects of some drugs not infrequently limit mobility. Occasionally, an old person can suddenly 'go off his feet' and for no obvious reason become bedfast. These cases are analogous to the 'failure to thrive' syndrome in infants and the cause may be equally difficult to find. Sometimes diseases such as chest infection are responsible. More than one pathology may contribute to immobility and such conditions as obesity and anaemia often exacerbate the problem. Extreme old age itself can influence movement (disuse atrophy), although it is often surprising how spry many 90-year-old people can be.

Skeletal Causes – Bone

The principal cause of reduced mobility from bone disease is pain. This may be severe and persistent or merely fleeting. The main diseases producing bone pain are osteoporosis, osteomalacia, Paget's disease and malignancy. Leeming[1] calculates that a GP with a list of 3,000 patients will have 70 patients with osteoporosis, 20 patients with Paget's disease and he would see a case of osteomalacia once every two to eight years. Much research has recently been carried out on bone physiology and there is rapidly expanding knowledge of the disordered metabolism behind many of these diseases, but despite these advances, practical treatment of bone disease has not in fact significantly improved.

Osteoporosis. This is basically a benign condition associated with a generalised loss or thinning of the bone, the fundamental matrix however, remaining normal. Symptoms and signs are usually not present until structural failure occurs, which may begin in women as early as 50, but in men not perhaps until after 65 years. It shows itself in loss of height and bowing due to thinning of the vertebral bodies and may be associated with fractures, particularly of the lower forearm in women and the neck of the femur in both sexes (after the age of 70). Compression fractures also occur in the lumbar vertebrae, giving localised backache. Elderly women seem to suffer from the condition more frequently than men, possibly because of post-menopausal lack of oestrogen. Prolonged bed rest and steroid therapy may also be responsible. X-ray of the bones shows generalised rarefaction. Serum calcium, phosphorus and alkaline phosphatase levels are not affected.

The condition cannot be cured, but its incidence can be reduced by minimising bed rest in illness and being aware of the dangers of long-term steroid therapy. Diet, as always, should be adequate, especially in calcium and vitamin D. A pint of milk a day is a good prescription. Mobility should be encouraged. The use of anabolic steroids is debatable and there is no evidence that they increase the density of the bone. Pain is sometimes a feature and should be treated with analgesics.

Osteomalacia. This is quite a different condition which is characterised histologically by failure of new-formed bone to calcify and is due to a lack of vitamin D. This may be associated with dietary deficiency, malabsorption syndromes particularly following gastrectomy and poor vitamin D metabolism. In osteomalacia the serum calcium and phosphorus is often, though not invariably, reduced and the serum alkaline phosphatase level is raised in 80 per cent of cases. Interpreting the chemical findings in the blood is important. Venous blood should be taken from fasting patients to determine the levels of serum protein and blood urea, as these interfere with the calcium and phosphorus levels. A reduction in albumen level will lead to a reduction of serum calcium and a raised blood urea will cause a rise in serum phosphorus. Anaemia is also often present in these cases. Sometimes iliac crest biopsy is necessary to make a diagnosis. The clinical picture is characterised by weakness of the proximal limb muscles, causing difficulty in lifting the feet, which sometimes produces a waddling type of gait. Weakness of the shoulder muscles may also be present, making it difficult for the patient to raise the arms. Bone pain, especially in the back, thigh and shoulder region is usually present. The condition occurs less frequently than osteoporosis but diagnosis is important because it is easy to treat. Calciferol in the dose of 50,000 units or 1.25 mg daily for two weeks followed by tablets of calcium and vitamin D BPC in a dose of 1 tablet twice a day for 12 months is the usual therapy.[1] Treatment with large doses of calciferol should not be prolonged as this may produce hypercalcaemia followed by renal failure. To prevent a recurrence of osteomalacia and avoid its development in housebound patients, Leeming suggests that it is logical to give regular prophylactic vitamin D therapy to old people in a suitable tablet such as calcium with vitamin D BPC or vitamin A and D capsules BPC.[2] This is particularly valuable during the winter months. Very important too is the daily intake of milk. Small amounts of exposure to the sun are also beneficial and should be encouraged. Osteomalacia also occurs in patients with other bone disorders and it is perhaps justifiable to give doses of vitamin D to patients suffering from pain thought to be due to bone disease. Full biochemical investigations should, however, be performed first.

Paget's Disease. This produces bone deformity and increased fragility associated with excessive bone breakdown, followed by rapid replacement. It affects the skeleton in a patchy, symmetrical manner and is not generalised. Most commonly affected bones are the pelvis, the spine, femur, tibia, skull and clavicle. Because of the expansion and deformity which may occur in the affected bones, bowing is produced particularly in the femur and tibia. The disease has active and inactive phases and during the former, the affected bone may be warm to touch and the serum alkaline phosphatase level may be markedly raised. The serum calcium and phosphorus levels are, however, usually normal in mild cases. Heart failure is sometimes present due to the increased circulation through the affected bone, but is probably not very common amongst elderly patients. There may also be pain in the bone, but the greatest difficulty to the patient arises from the deformities which occur. Treatment of Paget's disease is perhaps not often necessary, apart from purely palliative measures. Recently, calcitonin given by injection once or twice a week has been found to be effective. This particularly relieves the pain and also produces a reduction in the serum alkaline phosphatase. It should therefore be considered when pain is severe or if there is reason to expect complications.

Malignant Disease. In old people, secondary deposits from primary lesions in the prostate, lung and breast occur in bones. Commonly affected are vertebral bodies, pelvis, femur and humerus. Multiple myeloma is not a rarity in old age and may cause bone pain. The serum calcium level may be normal or raised, but the serum phosphorus and alkaline phosphatase concentrations are usually normal. X-ray films are necessary to make a full diagnosis. Renal failure may be a complication of multiple myeloma and Bence Jones protein may be found in the urine. Erythrocyte sedimentation rate is usually high and the serum globulin level is commonly raised. Carcinoma of the prostate producing secondaries usually causes a rise in the serum acid phosphatase level. The treatment of malignant conditions is basically that of general cancer but doses of radiation to the affected bony parts often prove to be temporarily beneficial.

Other Skeletal Causes. Other causes of bone pain restricting mobility are recent injuries, undiagnosed fractures, or the effect of poorly healed fractures causing deformity. These can sometimes be pathological and can occur with any of the conditions mentioned above. Increasing pain raises the possibility of this type of fracture. A rare cause of bone pain in elderly patients is the subperiosteal haematoma associated with scurvy.

Skeletal Causes – Joints

Osteoarthritis. This is an extremely common condition in old age and its incidence may be as high as 80 per cent. It is due to degenerative changes in the joints. The clinical features are limited movement with pain and some wasting of the surrounding muscles. Stiffness and deformity of the joints is found and crepitus may be felt on movement. Heberden's nodes are a characteristic finding, particularly in old age. It is often associated with obesity and the common joints to be involved are the hips and knees. Parts of the spine are also affected. X-ray changes are characteristic although not all patients with X-ray changes complain about joint pains. Treatment involves weight reduction and the use of anti-inflammatory drugs such as aspirin, paracetamol, phenylbutazone and ibuprofen. Many preparations of aspirin are available and the various enteric-coated varieties are better tolerated in old age. Benoral can be useful, particularly in its liquid form. Physiotherapy as heat and massage is helpful and many old people seem to derive benefit from massaging the joint with olive oil or some other bland agent. Rubifacients have also their adherents but it is hard to see how they really have any therapeutic effect and, because of possible skin damage, are best avoided. Despite this, many old people enjoy and believe in the therapeutic value of good rubbing bottle.

Intra-articular injections of cortisone can occasionally be used to relieve the acute pain of inflamed joints. Surgical treatment is possible and hip replacements have been undertaken in quite extreme old age. Osteotomy, which is an operation to change the stress forces on diseased joints, may bring relief from pain. When mobility is severely restricted as a result of osteoarthritic joints of the lower limbs, walking aids such as tripods may be necessary. Bed rest should be kept to an absolute minimum in these cases because of the increased risk of contractures.

Rheumatoid Arthritis. This condition can be present in an old person as a residue of illness suffered in earlier years, and is usually in an inactive form. It can also have its onset in old age. The disease consists of polyarthritis, particularly involving the small joints of the hands and feet, and the distribution tends to be symmetrical as distinct from the asymmetrical distribution of osteoarthritis. There is a proliferative inflammation of the synovial membrane and this results in irreversible damage to the joint capsule and articular cartilage. As it is a constitutional illness, there may also be loss of weight, anaemia and generalised debility. Treatment is on the lines indicated for osteoarthritis, but more specific anti-rheumatoid therapy (cortico-steroids, or gold injection for example) is sometimes used.

Other Joint Causes. There are rarer forms of arthritis, such as septic arthritis, psoriatic arthritis and gout, which cause painful joints in old people and hence reduce mobility.

Muscle

Many minor muscular lesions, such as *fibrositis*, can cause trouble for old people. These conditions can be effectively treated by simple analgesics and heat. An illness which affects elderly people particularly is *poly-myalgia rheumatica.* This is more common in women and associated with pain and stiffness in the neck, spreading to the shoulder muscles and also the gluteal and thigh muscles. The patient may also have generalised symptoms such as headaches, sweating and anorexia. The condition is sometimes associated with a temporal arteritis and in both the erythrocyte sedimentation rate is raised. The illness lasts for a few months and is likely to be recurrent. Analgesics will relieve the symptoms, but the treatment basically is by steroids; sometimes as much as 20 mg of Prenisolone three times daily may be required. The dose is then reduced according to the level of the ESR or plasma viscosity and the relief of symptoms.

Feet

The condition of the feet of old people is important as disorders easily impede mobility. Bunions associated with hallux valgus may be extremely painful, as are corns and callouses. Toe-nail deformity may make walking extremely difficult. Recently, the prevalence of fungal infection of the feet of patients in geriatric wards has been highlighted and in a sample of patients, almost all had positive cultures for certain fungal organisms. Perhaps it would be a good idea if chiropodists dealing with old people also looked for and treated any fungal infections. In institutions, laundry methods should treat stockings with suitable disinfectants. Disposable bath mats are also helpful in preventing this type of infection.

Neurological Causes

The various defects produced as a result of cerebrovascular disease are perhaps the commonest neurological cause of immobility and these are described in Chapter 16. Apart from these, there are two conditions which commonly produce mobility defects. These are Parkinson's disease and lower motor neurone disease.

Parkinson's Disease. Dr James Parkinson, who was an East London general practitioner, first described the disease in 1817. He called it 'the shaking palsy' but it is also sometimes known as 'paralysis agitans'. It is probable that degenerative changes in the blood vessels, supplying the basic basal ganglia in the brain, cause the disease, but it can occur after encephalitis. Parkinsonism is a rather general term used to describe the symptoms of Parkinson's disease and these symptoms can be caused by certain drugs.

The condition is characterised by akinesia (lack of movement), rigidity and tremor. The face shows a mask-like appearance and dementia may be an associated condition. The shuffling gait consisting of a few small steps and the tendency to lean forward, with difficulty in stopping, is frequently seen. Generalised clumsiness is often present, with difficulty in dressing and undressing a marked feature. The rigidity may be severe and the cogwheel effect of a series of small jerks when moving the elbow may be demonstrated. The tremor starts in the hand and is coarse, becoming less when a voluntary movement is undertaken, and disappears during sleep.

Major advances have taken place in the treatment of Parkinson's disease and drug therapy has become very much a possibility. Complex physiological principles are involved, based on the acetyl choline-dopamine balance in the brain. The dosage, side-effects and indications of the various drugs used need to be known and these have been excellently described in some textbooks of geriatrics and phamacology. Surgical treatment is also a possibility but seems not to be widely practised in elderly patients.

Motor Neurone Disease. This is characterised by wasting of the muscles of all four limbs. Fasciculation or fine movements in the muscles can be seen and the reflexes are brisk. The weakness associated with the muscle wasting can sometimes become severe, and can lead to considerable difficulty in patient movement. This can be particularly burdensome when the mental state remains unimpaired and the patient who has previously been able to look after himself or herself and even drive a car finds it extremely frustrating to be limited by muscular weakness. The condition can last for some time but will eventually result in the patient being unable to care for herself. The tongue and throat muscles can be affected, giving rise to difficulties with salivation, swallowing and nutrition.

Management of Immobility

It can be seen that there are many causes of immobility. Some physical ones have been described and many mental illnesses in old age can reduce the patient's ability to move around. There must be motivation to move out of the house or at least out of the chair. Sometimes an inconveniently placed house can psychologically deter an old person from making the effort to venture outside.

Management has to take all these factors into account and it is important that full medical examination and correct diagnosis should be made to detect underlying conditions. Physical illness must be treated, sometimes by the use of specific drugs as with thyroid replacement in cases of hypothyroidism, but also in conditions such as osteoarthritis by pain-relieving drugs. Chiropody may be all that is necessary in some circumstances, but occasionally full rehabilitation services may be needed to mobilise the patient. The provision of aids, appliances and modifications to the house are often helpful, particularly as part of a general programme of physiotherapy. Stimulating an old person mentally by encouraging interest in an outside activity or a hobby can change a housefast isolate once more into a member of the community. Change in housing can sometimes help. For instance, a lady of 80 with osteoarthritic knees was rendered housefast because the stairs of her first-floor flat were too hazardous. Getting on and off buses was also painful and she lacked courage to attempt a journey to the shops. Transfer to ground-floor accommodation near the shopping precinct enabled her to become mobile and independent once more.

Falls

Falls are a major hazard of old age and a common cause of injury and sometimes death. A.N.G. Clarke, when studying falls, found that nearly three-quarters of them occurred in or near the patient's home and about one-fifth further afield.[3] These latter take place almost exclusively near roads, particularly on pavements, kerbs and pedestrian crossings, where distraction by traffic or uneven surfaces are commonly causal factors.

Getting on and off buses can also be a hazard. The remainder of falls take place usually in welfare homes or hospital and it is less common for them to occur in such places as churches, shops and places of work.

Clarke describes three main types of fall mechanism.

Accidental falls: here the event is determined by environmental factors only, for example, slipping on an icy surface or tripping over a rug or a mat.

Symptomatic falls: here the cause is due to factors within the patient and can result from either fits or faints. In this group are also falls caused by dizziness or light-headedness.

Mixed type falls: here both environmental and patient factors are combined.

Causes of Falls

Of the accidental variety there are many possible causes; they include trips, slips and being knocked over by a vehicle or another person. Symptomatic falls can be caused, as stated above, by fits or faints. Grand mal type epileptic fits might be due to pre-existing idiopathic epilepsy or to cerebrovascular disease, intra-cranial tumour, trauma or hypoglycaemia. Fainting attacks without the characteristics of a fit may be due to transient ischaemic attack, cardiac infarction, a Stokes-Adams attack or postural hypotension. Another cause is the so-called 'drop attack' whose nature is still rather obscure. Characteristically, in these attacks, the patient, most commonly a woman, falls suddenly because without warning the legs go weak and flaccid. There is no loss of consciousness but the unsteadiness of the legs often persists for some time. Falls also occur at night when the patient is wandering. These may be due to postural hypotension occurring when a person gets out of bed quickly, following a sudden urge to pass urine. A patient may be confused at night because of too-heavy sedation or restless because of too little sedation. Both circumstances can lead to nocturnal wanderings and cause falls. Over-use of alcohol by old people, a problem which is perhaps increasing, can also be contributory. Patients with general debility and frailness are more likely to fall, particularly if they also suffer from some disability which impedes mobility, such as arthritis or Parkinson's disease, especially when this is combined with poor vision. Falls are also more likely after a period in bed because of illness.

It seems that there is a physiological decline in postural control with advancing age and falls are often associated with impaired balance. Old people are unable to correct themselves once they have stumbled, and there is a higher percentage of falls from causes other than tripping in patients over 75 years.

Management

Management of acute fall depends of course on the injuries sustained. If possible, an eye-witness account of the episode should be obtained so that if there is a possibility that the fall was due to a fit, investigation can be undertaken. This could be very extensive if all the possible causes of a fit in an old person were to be eliminated and common sense is necessary when deciding what tests to undertake. Help from a consultant geriatrician is usually to be recommended. Again, when the cause of the fall has been a faint of some type, a search for possible disease causes should be made. Some of these conditions can be treated and it is important that this should be done if possible.

It is often necessary to look at the patient's social circumstances. Safety in the home must be assessed and the arrangement of the patient's living area may need adjustment. Sometimes it is necessary where a person is having frequent falls and is living alone, to arrange transfer to welfare accommodation or warden-supervised housing.

Prevention of Falls

The aim should be if possible to prevent falls. Clarke lists simple ways of approaching the problem and these are summarised here.[4]

1. Removal of Hazards in the Home. In many instances these are obvious, but particular attention should be paid to loose rugs, carpets with holes and uneven surfaces. A good standard of lighting is essential and high wattage bulbs should be used. Handrails may be fitted to aid the old person's movement. All fires should be protected by fire-guards.

2. Preservation of Good Health and Confidence. When a patient has had a fall, assessment is necessary so that treatable conditions can be remedied. Poor vision should be corrected if possible. Careful rehabilitation after illness or injury should reduce the possibility of further accident.

3. Wearing of Appropriate Footwear. Rubber and crepe soles are unsatisfactory in wet and icy conditions. Non-slip or leather soles are preferable.

4. Special Care Outdoors. In winter, when conditions are bad, high-risk persons should remain indoors. If it is necessary to go out, they should be accompanied and routes chosen where there is likely to be the least danger from distraction by traffic. Busy roads should be crossed on pedestrian crossings. Shopping should be carried in a wheeled container. Care should be taken when boarding and alighting from public transport. A careful watch should be kept for uneven surfaces and care at kerbs observed.

5. Awareness of the Dangers of Sudden Changes in Posture. Patients should be careful when getting in and out of bed or chairs and instructed to do this slowly.

6. Monitoring of Night Sedation. Careful attention is needed to the level of night sedation prescribed for an old person, since this may be more a cause of falls than a help. Indeed, all drug therapy for patients with falls should be reviewed. Night sedation should, however, be adequate so that nocturnal wanderings are avoided.

It is obviously essential to identify patients who are at risk of falling. Screening old people at clinics for the elderly can help and note can be made of patients with a history of falling. Preventive measures can then be instituted and patients educated about the various safety precautions.

Notes

1. James T. Leeming, 'Skeletal Disease in the Elderly' *British Medical Journal*, vol.4 (1973), pp.472-4.
2. Ibid.
3. A.N.G. Clarke, 'Falls in Old Age', *Modern Geriatrics*, vol.2, no.6 (1972), pp.332-6.
4. Ibid.

Further Reading

Monica Cheale, 'Fits, Faints and Falls in the Elderly', *Update*, vol.8, no.3 (1974), pp.311-20.

Nicholas Coni, William Davison and Stephen Webster, *Lecture Notes on Geriatrics* (Oxford and Edinburgh, Blackwell Scientific Publications, 1977).

15 DIABETES MELLITUS

Elderly diabetic patients may be long-established diabetics, or may have recently acquired the disease in its late onset form. The prevalence of diabetes in old age is difficult to ascertain, partly because of the differing significance attached by experts to various levels of blood sugar in elderly patients. It is generally agreed that a fasting blood sugar of over 130 mg per 100 ml (7.2 m mol/litre) or a blood sugar level, 2 hours after 50 g of glucose by mouth has been administered, of over 200 mg per 100 ml (11.1 m mol/litre) indicates diabetes and the patient should be treated accordingly. In people with lower degrees of elevation it has been suggested by Ferguson Anderson that treatment might be beneficial in reducing the specific complications of diabetes, and also the frequency of arterial disease.[1]

Up to a quarter of the population of patients over 75 years old have abnormal glucose tolerance tests,[2] but many of these patients are without glycosuria.[3] Diabetes mellitus has been shown to be a possible undiagnosed condition in the elderly and in a survey of patients of over 75 years old in general practice the prevalence of diabetes mellitus was 5 per cent and half of it was previously unreported.[4]

The classical symptoms of thirst and polyuria are relatively uncommon in the elderly although weight loss and pruritis may give the first hint of developing diabetes. Pruritis valvae and balanitis are often present. A patient developing incontinence or bed-wetting should be suspected of the condition and again, these are often early symptoms. Diabetes may also present as one of its complications. These include vascular disease due to arteriosclerosis either as coronary thrombosis or ischaemic disease of the lower limb. This latter, when combined with diabetic neuropathy which often causes loss of sensation in the feet, can cause infected ulcers and eventually gangrene, and is a serious complication. An old person with a predisposition to infection should be suspected of having diabetes. Another complication which sometimes presents is renal failure. Keto acidosis is rare in old people but any confused or comatosed elderly patient should be suspected of having the disease, particularly if he is dehydrated. Abdominal pain may be a striking feature of diabetes in old age and often develops in people not previously known to be diabetic.[5] A mild case of late-onset diabetes is sometimes found at a preventive screening clinic for the elderly by the finding of glycosuria. In these cases, estimation of the blood sugar level is necessary for diagnosis. Most clinics do routine blood sugar estimations and this is useful because a raised blood sugar may not be associated with glycosuria. Indeed the screening test for diabetes is a post-prandial blood sugar estimation. Late-onset cases are usually mild and the complications are more important than the actual disease.

Management

The problem facing the doctor once a diagnosis of late-onset diabetes has been made is how enthusiastically to treat the condition. Drugs should be kept as simple as possible because difficulties can arise from the patient's inability to adhere to complicated tablet regimes and the necessity for regular urine testing. Many old people, for economic reasons, live on a high carbohydrate diet and there are sometimes problems of adjustment. It is usually essential therefore to gain the help of some responsible relative or friend to supervise treatment. A general discussion will be necessary to explain the nature of the problem and possible dangers, including the side-effects of drugs and complications of the disease.

Diet

Many cases of late-onset diabetes can be controlled by dietary measures. The diet should be simple, even if not quite correct, so that the patient can keep to it. He may easily lose heart coping with a detailed and complicated regime. The diet should be in the region of 100-200 g of carbohydrate daily, a good starting point for most elderly patients being about 140 g of carbohydrate. The modern tendency is to restrict fats and cholesterol a little because diabetes is associated with a raised serum cholesterol and diabetics have enough trouble with their arteries without encouraging atheroma. A very strict low-cholesterol diet is probably unnecessary but perhaps the patient should know which foods contain most cholesterol so that they avoid eating more than a reasonable 'small normal' amount of such things as eggs and cream. Dieticians are usually very helpful in advising about these problems and most Area Health Authorities now have dieticians who work in the community as well as in the hospital. Many of the patients are also obese and the total calorie intake should be restricted. Obesity can contribute to the arterial complications of diabetes.

Oral Hypoglycaemic Agents

Hypoglycaemic agents are now an established part of the treatment of diabetes in old age. They are useful in controlling the glycaemic symptoms of the condition but there is some doubt whether they reduce the incidence of such complications as vascular disease. Two questions need answering about the use of these agents. First, in what type of patient should they be given and secondly, which preparation is best in old age? The type of case where they are usually used is where diet alone does not control the diabetic symptoms. There are now a large number of hypoglycaemic agents available. They are of two types, the sulphonylureas (of which the most frequently used are probably chlorpropamide and tolbutamide) and the biguanides (metformin and phenformin). The most usual drug prescribed in old age is possibly chlorpropamide but there are some advantages in using tolbutamide in the first instance. It produces fewer gastro-intestinal side-effects and is shorter-acting, therefore reducing the likelihood of confusion induced by hypoglycaemia. The biguanides, particularly phenformin, should not be used for the aged as it is now recognised that they can predispose to lactic acid acidosis.

All hypoglycaemic agents can cause side-effects and these include gastro-intestinal upset, allergic skin reactions and, more seriously, blood dyscrasias such as leukopenia and thrombocytopenia. Hypoglycaemic agents also react with other drugs being taken. With chlorpropamide and possibly other sulphonylureas alcohol may interact and patients may experience hot flushes, giddiness, sickness and chest pain, 10-15 minutes after taking an alcoholic drink. It is necessary to warn patients about this possibility. Prolonged and unresponsive hypoglycaemia can occur with chlorpropamide in the elderly. Beta blockers make recognition of hypoglycaemia more difficult, so if taken with hypoglycaemic tablets or insulin, attacks of hypoglycaemia become much more troublesome. There may be an increased incidence of hypothyroidism in patients taking long-term sulphonylurea treatment. Patients with hepatic and renal failure should in theory not be given oral hypoglycaemic agents. Congestive heart failure is a special problem and the question is sometimes raised as to whether oral hypoglycaemic agents should be used with thiazide diuretics. In practice, if the patient is in a stable situation it is probably safe, providing (1) special caution is taken when starting treatment or changing the dose; (2) there is a constant awareness of the possibility that changes in the degree of failure, or reduction in hepatic or renal sufficiency, may change the diabetic state.

Insulin Treatment

Ferguson Anderson maintains that perhaps 20 per cent of elderly patients require insulin treatment.[6] This is better given as a single dose with a long-acting preparation such as PZI or Lente insulin. Injections for old people need supervision and it is probably inadvisable for them to inject themselves. This may, however, depend on the availability of community nurses. A careful change of site is necessary to avoid necrotic ulcers forming. If insulin is required in a newly established case, stabilisation is necessary in hospital because of the risks of hypoglycaemia. The danger of insulin therapy in an old person is the development of severe hypoglycaemia when meals are missed and incorrect doses are given. Clear instructions are absolutely essential. It is important to make sure that renal function is adequate. There is the possibility of a diabetic patient developing antibodies to insulin with a resulting increased risk of developing complications. To overcome this, new insulins have been introduced and when allergy or lipoatrophy are present, a change to one of these is indicated.

Treatment of Complications

Treatment of complications will be along the usual lines described in textbooks of medicine. At the earliest signs of difficulty, expert help should be sought and hypoglycaemic attacks should be treated in hospital. Chronic hypoglycaemia can easily be overlooked in the elderly since the only obvious symptoms may be mild confusion, shivering or sweating. These occur frequently in old age from other causes.

Follow-up

Regular follow-up is necessary to check the control of the diabetes and the possibility of complications. Foot problems should be avoided by regular visits to a chiropodist. There is also the problem of elderly diabetics who hold driving licences. The risks of hypoglycaemia are such that it is very important that advice should be given about eating before driving for any distance, and stopping frequently for snacks to step up the blood sugar level. If the patient finds that he does not have any warning of hypoglycaemia it is probably best to advise him to avoid driving altogether.

Usually a long-established diabetic will not require any alteration to his treatment as he grows older, but it is useful that he should attend a clinic regularly so that his condition may be monitored.

Notes and Further Reading

1. W. Ferguson Anderson, *Practical Management of the Elderly*, 2nd edition (Oxford and Edinburgh, Blackwell Scientific Publications, 1971).

2. W.J.H. Butterfield, *Proceedings of the Royal Society of Medicine*, no.57 (1964), p.196.

3. College of General Practitioners, 'Glucose Tolerance and Glycosuria in the General Population', *British Medical Journal*, vol.2 (1963), p.655.

4. E.I. Williams *et al.*, 'Sociomedical Study of Patients over 75 in General Practice', *British Medical Journal*, vol.2 (1972), pp.445-8.

5. M.F. Green, 'Endocrine Disorders in the Elderly', *British Medical Journal*, vol.1 (1974), pp.232-6.

6. Anderson, *Practical Management of the Elderly*.

16 STROKE

Stroke is a common condition and is the main cause of death in this country after heart disease and cancer. Each year, nearly 2 in every 1,000 of the population will suffer from a stroke. Amongst the elderly, the incidence rises steeply and a high proportion occur in people over 65 years of age. Strokes are also responsible for considerable residual disability. Among the survivors it can be expected that one-third will recover, one-third will be completely dependent and the remaining third will have some impairment in functional ability. Although perhaps half of those who suffer from a stroke will die in the first few weeks, it can be seen that many persons suffering from the effects of the condition will be present in the community.

Underlying Basic Pathology

The term 'stroke' is perhaps loosely applied to describe the clinical manifestation of two distinct happenings in the cerebro-vascular system. These are sometimes jointly referred to as 'cerebro-vascular accidents' (CVA). They consist either of a haemorrhage from a blood vessel or a blockage (sometimes called occlusion) in it, caused usually by a clot or thrombus, but could also be due to an embolus arising, sometimes in the heart, sometimes in the carotid and cerebro-vascular arteries. This latter produces death of the part of the brain supplied by the particular artery affected. The area of destroyed tissue is called an infarction. Thus cerebral thrombosis or occlusion produces cerebral infarction and these are part of the same process. The position and extent of the infarction determines the various clinical pictures. Haemorrhage from a cerebral artery causes infusion of blood into the surrounding brain tissues and causes damage in this way, as well as by cutting off or reducing the blood supply to the parts supplied by the artery.

Within the group of cerebro-vascular incidents (as opposed to accidents) are episodes of so-called transient ischaemic attacks (TIAs). The underlying cause is different and consists of a reduction in the blood supply to the brain which is only a short duration. This is due to temporary blockage of parts of the cerebral circulation by micro-emboli of dislodged platelets arising from atheromatous plaques situated at, for instance, the bifurcation of the common carotid artery, the vertebro-basilar artery, or in some cases, the heart itself. The dislodgement of these emboli may be precipitated by a fall in the blood pressure from such causes as coronary thrombosis. Anaemia, hypoglycaemia, renal and hepatic failure can also help to cause transient ischamic attacks. Obstruction of the blood supply to the brain by cervical spondylosis may also be contributory.

Clinical Presentation

1. Transient Ischaemic Attacks

These are important as they may herald a full cerebral thrombosis. They are treatable and it may be possible to take action to avoid more serious trouble. The clinical findings can vary and depend on the source of the micro-emboli. Those arising in the carotid artery may be associated with eye symptoms such as hemianopia or even complete blindness, and also with limb weakness, which is usually unilateral. Speech defects may also occur. Sometimes a murmur may be audible over the carotid artery. When the source of the micro-emboli is the vertebro-basilar arterial system, the symptoms include dizziness, eye symptoms such as double vision, or again, complete loss of sight, limb weakness (which is often bilateral) and speech difficulty. Memory disturbances may also be a feature. Vertebro-basilar attacks are said to have a better prognosis and rarely proceed to full stroke. In practice, however, it is clinically often difficult to separate these two types. A careful examination of the heart may reveal disease which may be the source of micro-emboli from this organ. Full recovery, however, takes place within a few minutes and certainly within 24 hours, although the attacks may be recurrent.

2. Complete Stroke

The clinical presentation of a complete stroke can be very complex and the effects can range widely from the severe to the mild. Early symptoms of headache, unsteadiness and sensations of weakness can be experienced by the patient. These can often be remembered clearly and described dramatically at a later period. In the acute stage, consciousness may be lost and deep coma ensue; in other cases the patient may remain lucid throughout the episode. A whole range of neurological deficits can occur, but most commonly, the person is left with a hemiplegia, together with weakness of the facial muscles and sometimes a speech defect. Other conditions may be present at the same time as a stroke and some, such as hypertension or a fibrillating heart, may have led directly to the attack. It is often impossible to distinguish clearly between cerebral thrombosis and cerebral haemorrhage; the latter is most likely to be the underlying event if there is a pre-existing hypertension and is more likely to occur in a younger individual. In both haemorrhage and embolus, the onset of the stroke is likely to be sudden.

Management

Several immediate actions may be needed when faced with a person suffering from a cerebral accident. Urgent first aid is often necessary and breathing difficulty may make it essential to ensure a clear airway. False teeth should be removed and the inhalation of vomit avoided by positioning the patient on his side. There is usually little doubt as to the diagnosis but if the doctor is early on the scene, there may be difficulty in deciding whether someone has suffered from a full stroke or merely a transient ischaemic attack. Sometimes the problem is solved by rapid improvement of symptoms but in any event, if the general condition of the patient is satisfactory, the doctor can reasonably wait a little before making a final diagnosis. Sometimes, cases present with increased intracranial pressure as demonstrated by the presence of papilloedema; intravenous administration of dexamethazone or frusemide may then be necessary as a first aid measure. Other conditions apart from cerebrovascular accident may produce raised pressure, and the doctor should enquire for a history of injury and consider the possibility of a resulting sub-dural haematoma. A history of headache, especially in the presence of papilloedema, may indicate the presence of a cerebral tumour. Infection may also produce a similar clinical picture and a note should be taken of a raised temperature and neck stiffness to exclude the presence of, for instance, meningitis. Many other conditions can also mimic cerebro-vascular accident in old age and these can include epilepsy, migraine, cardiac conditions, Stokes-Adams attacks and hypoglycaemia.

All these possibilities should be borne in mind by the doctor when making the initial assessment, but following this, it will be necessary to make the often difficult decision as to whether to admit the patient to hospital. In cases of transient ischaemic attacks, most GPs would be prepared to treat the condition at home, but with complete stroke, the decision is not as clear. Some will say that all stroke patients should be admitted to hospital and although this may be theoretically correct, there are others who are prepared to treat mild cases at home. There are several factors to be considered. The patient's clinical condition is often all-important. Mild hemiplegias with rapidly recovering movement may be suitable for home care. Sometimes, in the case of a very old patient where detailed investigation is contra-indicated, it is better to keep him at home and thus avoid the stresses, both mental and physical, of being transferred by ambulance to the new environment of a hospital. Extension of a stroke can indeed sometimes be precipitated by such movement. If death is imminent and the condition obviously terminal, it is more humane to nurse the patient at home and hospital admission should be avoided.

The nature and extent of extra-cerebral disease also needs assessing and such conditions as heart failure and broncho-pneumonia concurrently present will indicate hospital admission. A previous history of stroke may mean transfer, as also when there is impaired consciousness. If the general health of the patient was good before the stroke and he was not suffering from hypertension, it is reasonable to consider home management.

Another important consideration is whether adequate nursing is available. Will the relatives be able to look after the patient and are there suitable bedroom facilities? Family reaction to strokes can vary; some insist that the patient be admitted to hospital, and some insist on the reverse. Hospital admission becomes essential, however, when constant and complex treatment is likely to be necessary. Doubt may sometimes exist as to whether the condition is due to thrombosis or to treatable haemorrhage. In these cases, full investigation is indicated, including examination of the cerebro-vascular fluid and, if available, computer-assisted axial tomography by EMI scanning. Neurosurgical treatment is available for cerebro-vascular episodes due to haemorrhage and this is of course the argument for hospital admission of all stroke cases, so that a full investigation can be carried out. This really is more important for younger subjects suffering from a stroke caused by a possible sub-arachnoid haemorrhage. This is a special type of brain haemorrhage which can be helped surgically. In the elderly, however, the possibility of such neurosurgical intervention occurs much less frequently. There are regional variations in the facilities for investigation and only certain areas have special stroke units. When these are available, a fine balance of judgement is necessary when considering the question of whether to admit an old person to hospital or proceed with home care.

Treatment of transient ischaemic attacks usually involves two to three days of rest and a gradual resumption of activity within a week. Any possible underlying cause, such as anaemia, drug misuse or hypoglycaemia should be treated and this will mean doing investigations such as full blood count, blood sugar level, chest X-ray and ECG. Temporal arteritis is sometimes a cause of transient ischaemic attack and ESR or blood viscosity should be done to check for this. Serological studies can be included in the investigations to exclude rare cases of neurosyphilis. Blood pressure should be monitored and the diastolic level kept below 100 mm of mercury by using anti-hypertensive agents if necessary. There are arguments in favour of full hospital investigation of patients who have suffered from a transient ischaemic attacks because it may be possible to prevent further episodes and particularly the onset of a full cerebral accident by surgical procedures such as endarterectomy. The question of anti-coagulation on a long-term basis will also have to be considered. In younger patients these are probably mandatory but in the elderly, careful thought needs to be taken as to whether the procedures are worthwhile. Full consideration with consultants in geriatric medicine is advisable under these circumstances.

Management of a case of full stroke at home involves three things: medical care, nursing care and rehabilitation. Medically, treatment of any underlying or associated illness needs undertaking and will usually be straightforward, but treatment of the actual stroke sometimes presents dilemmas. Anti-coagulants are obviously contra-indicated at home but the use of steroids and diuretics as cerebral decongestants must be considered. There is also the problem as to whether to treat hypertension. The patient may be already on treatment and this should be continued. In the early stages of the stroke, it is probably unwise to reduce a raised blood pressure, but later, if the diastolic level is over 120 mm of mercury, it may be necessary to use hypotensive or diuretic agents. The cardiac and renal state must be carefully assessed before embarking on this treatment. Generally in old age, hypotensive drugs should be used cautiously, particularly in established cerebro-vascular disease. The presence of cerebral dementia contra-indicates their use completely.

Nursing care will involve the usual attention to such things as general washing, cleaning, toileting, maintenance of adequate fluid levels and dietary advice. Lifting paralysed patients up and down the bed requires care to avoid shoulder sub-luxation and is usually a two-handed task. The head should be elevated to reduce cerebral oedema. The period of bed rest should be reduced to as short a time as possible in order to reduce the risk of thrombosis in the veins of the calf muscles, hypostatic pneumonia, joint contractures and pressure sores.

Rehabilitation will be necessary if the patient is going to make a good functional recovery and should start at the beginning of the illness.

The stages of rehabilitation have been described in Chapter 11. It might be that the physiotherapy fails to influence the neurological outcome but nevertheless, the patient's ability to cope with daily living can probably be improved by exercises which improve general fitness and enable other working muscles to compensate. The success of this type of rehabilitation may be better at home than in hospital.

When the acute stage has passed and life is preserved, the aim of management must be not only to enable the patient to make as full a functional recovery as possible, but also to avoid a recurrence of further strokes. This latter will probably mean investigations on the lines suggested for transient ischaemic attacks and consultant opinion is once more necessary. Full recovery cannot, however, be expected in all cases of stroke, and finally the health care team is left with patients where residual damage is present, who were either managed at home in the first place or have been discharged from hospital. The full resources of rehabilitation services are necessary to enable this type of patient to adjust to the disability and the inevitably restricted life-style. The patient's psychological adjustment to this situation also needs attention, and the family's attitude to this needs to be discussed, particularly as this may involve considerable social adaptation. Help from all members of the primary health care team should be forthcoming, particularly to reassure the patient that he has not been forgotten once the initial episode has been successfully overcome. There are many severely handicapped hemiplegics who have benefited from successful rehabilitation in the early stages, but who regress once this is finally withdrawn. The family are left eventually with most of the responsibility and they often need help, particularly when speech has been affected, and communication with a patient is difficult. Valerie Eaton-Griffiths describes an interesting experiment in Buckinghamshire, where volunteers were recruited to visit patients in the post-stroke phase in order to help them through this difficult time.[1] Home visits were arranged and a club was formed in the village hall. It was found that this 'good neighbour scheme' maintained by quite untrained volunteers was welcomed by both patients and families. This undoubtedly is a very good example of support that can be given by interested people, and is particularly valuable where no more benefit is going to be possible from medical attention.

Finally, how possible is it to prevent stroke or recurrence of stroke in elderly people? This is uncertain but some precursor conditions such as diabetes, obesity and heart failure can be treated effectively and should be identified. There is now growing evidence that a diastolic pressure of over 105 mm of mercury is abnormal in old age. It is possible that by treating patients with this level or over, using diuretics or beta blockers, strokes may be prevented. The place of long term anti-coagulants and arterial surgery in old age remains, however, still speculative.

Notes

1. Valerie Eaton-Griffiths, 'Volunteer Scheme for Dysphasia and Allied Problems in Stroke Patients', *British Medical Journal*, vol.3 (1975), pp.633-5.

Further Reading

John Grabinar, 'A Case for the Conservative Treatment of Strokes', *Update*, vol.11, no.9 (October 1975), pp.899-904.

M. Keith Thompson, 'A Case for the Active Treatment of Strokes', *Update*, vol.11, no.10 (November 1975), pp.1001-15.

17 SPECIAL MEDICAL PROBLEMS

In this chapter four subjects are included which often need to be discussed when seeing a patient at a clinic for the elderly. Failing vision or deafness frequently need attention. Many old people have had the same glasses for a considerable time and retesting is long overdue. A discussion of hearing aids is also welcomed. It is usually the health visitor who brings up the subject of nutritition and it is she also who might be aware of hypothermia risk situations.

Nutrition in the Elderly

Both doctors and social workers may be involved in the nutritional state of old people, and it is sometimes necessary to assess whether they are getting adequate nourishment and also to advise on the proper food intake. This is particularly true of those who may be too apathetic to cook proper meals, such as the very old, those living alone and the disabled. It is useful, therefore, to have some idea of how to assess nutrition and to have an appreciation of the causes of poor food intake so that they may be identified and avoided.

It is not easy to be dogmatic about the ideal level of nutrition and there are considerable differences in the needs of people in general for energy and nutrients. These variations persist into old age. Body size, sex and physical activity are all factors which influence need. The quality of the food and the ease with which it is absorbed are also relevant. However, with increasing age, there is a gradual decrease in physical activity and a decline in metabolism at rest. It is to be expected, therefore, that the food intake of old people will be reduced and this ideally should be evenly distributed throughout the diet. Under these circumstances, where there is a balanced reduction of the various foods, malnutrition should not occur. This is probably true for most of the elderly people but there are circumstances where faulty nutrition may be present.

How prevalent is malnutrition? Early surveys tended to find a fair amount of inadequate food intake and established cases of, for instance, scurvy, were sometimes encountered. Many of these studies were on patients admitted to hospital and perhaps were not typical of the elderly population in the community. The now classical studies of Bransby and Osborne, which formed part of the Sheffield study, indicated that perhaps old people in the community were coping well with their domestic responsibilities, although there were wide variations in the consumption of particular foods.[1] More recent studies, such as those of Exton-Smith and Stanton, have found that although food intake decreases with advancing age, many of the elderly subjects managed to eat a varied diet.[2] A nutritional survey of the elderly carried out by the DHSS found some overt malnutrition, but not much; the report stresses, however, that many are vulnerable and the margin of safety may be slight.[3] There is obviously the need to identify and treat individuals at risk before disability or sudden catastrophe overtakes them so that malnutrition may be avoided.

Clinical Assessment of Nutrition

Assessment of the nutritional status of an old person is important but difficult. It is sometimes necessary for a doctor or health visitor to find out whether a person is getting enough food and the information available for doing this is often unreliable and vague. Under these circumstances, one has to rely on physical examination to determine whether the patient is well nourished. This may also present difficulties as specific signs of malnutrition may be totally lacking. Weight loss is an important feature but examples of serious under-nutrition with severe weight loss are rarely encountered apart from in some cases of senile dementia. More moderate weight loss may be due to under-nutrition, but interpretation is difficult as it may be due to several other causes. Ageing itself results in reduction in body mass and concomitant disease can also influence weight.

Clinically, poor nutrition can show itself in general apathy and lassitude, and unexplained anaemia may well point to an inadequate diet. Some of the factors likely to lead to sub-nutrition may be present and these will be discussed shortly. Reduction in subcutaneous fat and skinfold thickness is sometimes regarded as a sign of poor nutrition. There may also, apart from reduction in calorie and protein intake, be an inadequate supply of vitamins in the diet and there is evidence to suggest that this can occur in up to half the elderly population. Although the lack of one vitamin, such as vitamin C, may occur alone, the signs of frank deficiency and disease are usually due to several different food factors being absent. When assessing the nutritional status, it is therefore essential to take note of any possible vitamin deficiency. Old men living alone may sometimes show signs of vitamin C deficiency; small haemorrhages may be the only sign and these may be seen particularly in the gums and under the tongue. Confirmation can be obtained by assessing the level of ascorbic acid within the white blood cells and platelets. Early diagnosis of osteomalacia caused by vitamin D deficiency should be made biochemically (see page 176) because when X-ray changes have occurred, the situation is often too late.

Factors Affecting Nutrition

Physical changes occur in old age which can contribute to a reduction in food intake. The teeth, for instance, are often lost and although mastication is possible without them, it becomes more difficult. Dentures may be unsatisfactory and might limit the choice of foods. Loss of taste and smell can reduce the appetite in old people. The flow of saliva also decreases as age advances, and this may make mastication more difficult. Oesophageal and gastric mobility may be impaired and gastric secretion reduced. This may affect food absorption as also may the presence of a previous partial gastrectomy.

General physical debility is an important cause of under-nutrition. The presence of such diseases as heart failure, chronic infection and arthritis can decrease an old person's interest in food. Some drugs may interfere with the absorption of certain vitamins, notably folic acid. These include phenytoin, phenylbutazone and nitrofurantoin. The mental state of an old person may also influence his dietary intake. It is likely to be reduced in patients with depression or early dementia. Sometimes dietary fads persist and are exaggerated in old age. A gastric diet may be maintained for far longer than is necessary and actually contribute to under-nutrition. On the other hand, diet may be well maintained despite quite severe behaviour disorder. Alcoholism may be present and be responsible for a loss of appetite, a fact which is often hidden from the doctor and relatives.

Various environmental factors can influence the food intake of old people. The actual physical preparation of food may be difficult. Kitchen layouts and cooking facilities may be unsuitable for the frail and disabled. Regular shopping for fresh supplies may not be undertaken because of reduced mobility. The author assessed the diet of 207 over-75-year-old people in 1970. One cooked meal per day was considered to be the lowest acceptable level of food intake and 28 were found to be below this. The numbers were relatively small, but it was found that inadequate diet was commonest in social classes 4 and 5 and amongst women between 80 and 90 years. Those living alone were also more likely to be poorly fed. It was found that the effective health of those on a poor diet was often diminished and also as an interesting footnote, that the mean haemoglobin level of patients on an inadequate diet was less than the group as a whole. These patients were not clinically malnourished but were obviously very vulnerable. How much was cause and effect is difficult to determine; perhaps once more a vicious circle is established where patients in poor health or with a low haemoglobin level become apathetic about food and reduced nutritional intake makes the condition worse.

Nutritional Requirements in Old Age

The Department of Health and Social Security has published a booklet on recommended intakes of nutrients for the UK.[4] The levels suggested for the elderly are given in Table 17.1. Not all commentators agree with these recommendations and they are not necessarily minimal requirements; nor are they much help in determining nutritional status, as lower levels may still be compatible with good health. Nevertheless, they are a reasonable guide and may be useful in planning diets for old people. The protein intake is relatively high and conforms with the currently held view that protein intake should provide 10 per cent of the energy requirement (Hyams).[5] Hyams suggests that a fat intake representing 20-25 per cent of the total calories is probably the most suitable for elderly people and an average intake of carbohydrate in a non-obese, non-diabetic subject would be 250-300 g per day. Adequate fibre in the diet is also now thought to be important.

Nutritional Help for the Elderly

Good dietary habits should start at an early age, and hopefully these will be continued into advanced years. Accepting that inadequate diet is a possibility, its early detection is important. It can easily be overlooked and it is necessary for doctors, health visitors and social workers to be constantly alert to the possibility. Certain groups already mentioned are vulnerable and need special attention. Screening clinics are helpful in recognising those at risk. Even making sure that old people have adequate dentures can reduce sub-nutrition and anaemia. Those who provide meals on wheels and supervise luncheon clubs can also recognise those whose appetites are poor or whose interest in food is deteriorating. Home helps are also valuable in helping old people to receive adequate nutrition. General education in the principles of nutrition should be part of the primary health care team's role, particularly in advocating the necesssity to eat fresh fruit and food rich in vitamins A and D, such as fish. Advances in technology have meant better packaging of food and much of it now is easy to prepare.

Table 17.1: Recommended Daily Intakes of Energy and Nutrients for the UK

Age Range	Occupational Category	Body weight	Energy		Protein	Thiamine	Ribo-flavine	Nicotic acid	Ascorbic acid	Vitamin A	Vitamin D	Calcium	Iron
		kg	kcal	mj	g	mg	mg	mg equivalents	mg	mg retinol equivts.	mg cholecal -ciferol	mg	mg
Men													
65 up to 75 years	Assuming a sedentary life	63	2,350	9.8	59	0.9	1.7	18	30	750	2.5	500	10
75 and over		63	2,100	8.8	53	0.8	1.7	18	30	750	2.5	500	10
Women													
55 up to 75 years	Assuming a sedentary life	53	2,050	8.6	51	0.8	1.3	15	30	750	2.5	500	10
75 and over		53	1,900	8.0	48	0.7	1.3	15	30	750	2.5	500	10

Source: *Recommended Intakes of Nutrients for the United Kingdom* DHSS Reports on Public Health and Medical Subjects, No.120.

Refrigerators and freezers have meant that storage is now possible for much longer periods and this may be invaluable when patients are incapacitated for a short period. Unfortunately, many old age pensioners do not have these facilities. The wisdom of adding extra vitamins to the diet either as pills or by fortifying foodstuffs is debatable. Excess of vitamins A and D, for instance, can be a hazard and in general, with a well balanced diet, additional vitamins should be unnecessary, except perhaps in winter for the housebound.

Old people with low incomes tend to buy cheaper foods and sometimes there is the dilemma of priorities as to whether money should be spent on other essentials such as fuel and clothing. Pensioners on Supplementary Benefit are entitled to additional allowances for special diets and they should be encouraged to apply for these, especially when such disabilities as a peptic ulcer or diabetes are present. To overcome any unsuitable domestic arrangements for cooking which are occasionally present, it is sometimes helpful for social workers to advise on alterations and special utensils. Easy access to ovens, shelves and storage units can enable a disabled person to cook for herself, when previously this was proving difficult. Teaching an old person to use these facilities is usually necessary. Meals on wheels and luncheon clubs are, of course, very important and great care is usually given to their nutritional content. Those living alone should be encouraged to use these facilities, especially if they can arrange to eat with others, as this often is a great stimulus to the appetite. Finally, there is the problem of obesity which, although rare in geriatric practice, occasionally occurs. This often shortens life expectancy and can aggravate many other problems. Help from hospital or community dieticians is often necessary to construct suitable diets.

Hypothermia

By definition, hypothermia is said to occur when the temperature of the body core (that is deep internal temperature) is less than 35°C (95°F). The condition was first described by Helen Duguid and her colleagues in 1961.[6] Of the 23 cases she described in her Scottish study, 22 were elderly. The Royal College of Physicians, in a survey carried out in 1965 involving 10 British hospitals, found a temperature of less than 35°C in 0.68 per cent of the admissions.[7] Although it is perhaps dangerous to extrapolate from these figures, it could be that several thousand people are admitted to hospital each year with a diagnosis of hypothermia. What the true incidence of the condition is in the community must at the moment be unknown, but it is probable that in winter it is not uncommon. Between four and five hundred deaths annually in Britain are said to be due to hypothermia, but this is probably a low estimate because the illness is not necessarily recognised or included in a death certificate.

Temperature

There are two aspects of temperature. There is the deep temperature, sometimes known as core temperature, around the vital organs within the centre of the body, which is maintained constantly despite variations in external conditions. But also, there is the temperature of skin and sub-cutaneous tissues, sometimes described as shell temperature and which varies with external temperature. In the elderly, the deep body temperature is about ½°C lower than in young people and this difference tends to increase as age advances.

Accurate recording of temperature is important when the possibility of hypothermia is present. Most clinical thermometers have as their lower reading 35°C. Special thermometers are therefore necessary to record low temperatures in old people. Care is needed to shake down the level of mercury sufficiently, for if this is not done the temperature of the body may be lower than the actual reading, as the mercury may not have risen at all. The usual method of oral measurement gives only the shell temperature. For assessment of core temperature, rectal measurement is necessary. Sometimes this is inconvenient, and some surveys have overcome this difficulty by measuring the temperature of the urine immediately after it has been passed. This is, however, outside the scope of normal clinical practice.

Heat Regulation

Maintenance of body temperature involves a fine balance between heat gain and heat loss. Physiologically a point is set within the body which indicates the temperature required and any difference is registered in the hypothalamus which sets off appropriate mechanisms for heat loss or gain. Peripheral cold reactors are stimulated when the body is exposed to cold and alternatively when overheating is the problem (as for instance when pyrogens are released during infections), the hypothalamus is stimulated to initiate heat controlling devices. Many factors affect these delicate mechanisms and an important one as far as the elderly are concerned is the relationship of mass to body surface. An animal with a large body mass, but a small body surface area, will have more difficulty in losing heat and special mechanisms will have to be introduced to allow this to happen. A thin, wasted old person on the other hand, with a large body surface, may have difficulty in conserving body heat and this may sometimes prove to be impossible. This may account partially for the impairment of temperature control which is seen in some old people.

Causes of Hypothermia

Although hypothermia is principally a condition of old age, it can also be found in babies and infants. Young people, such as climbers and yachtsmen who find themselves exposed for long periods to cold, wet conditions, can also suffer from hypothermia. The real cause is exposure to cold, but there are factors which exaggerate the effect of this. Impaired physiological maintenance of body temperature seems to be present in some people and this may make them more vulnerable. Many illnesses may be associated with impaired thermo-regulatory mechanisms, for instance myxoedema, hypo-pituitarism, diabetes, stroke, myocardial infarctions, infections and extensive skin lesions. Immobility produced by conditions such as arthritis, Parkinsonism and mental impairment can also be associated with hypothermia. Certain drugs, such as chlorpromazine (Largactil), diazepam (Valium) and, of course, alcohol can also be contributory. This is important when dealing with confused old people because sometimes the confusion may be due to hypothermia, and the use of phenothiazone tranquillisers (e.g. Largactil) may aggravate the hypothermic condition. The environment is also important. People living in cold, draughty houses, particularly those in high or exposed conditions, may be particularly vulnerable.

Clinical Manifestations

In an established case of hypothermia, the patient is obviously cold and this applies particularly to the abdomen and trunk. Strangely enough, he may not complain of cold. Other appearances have been described and include skin of a pale or pinkish colour which is sometimes puffy and creates a resemblance to myxoedema. The voice may also have a deeper tone than normal. The muscles may be rigid and the reflexes sluggish. Consciousness may be clouded and the patient may be drowsy. The pulse is usually slow and the blood pressure reduced. Breathing may be shallow and there may be signs of broncho-pneumonia, although hypothermia can mask this condition, and it is only when the patient is warmed that it becomes apparent. A situation seen in the community which is associated with hypothermia is where the old person has for some reason fallen out of bed. There may also be a fracture, particularly of the femur. The patient is usually unable to get back into bed and lies all night scantily clad in a cold bedroom. Discovery may not be for several hours and this type of exposure can rapidly lead to hypothermia. Hypothermia developing insidiously in old people is also very common and much more difficult to identify.

Treatment

It is possible to treat mild cases of hypothermia at home providing that there is adequate care available and that the social conditions in the house are reasonable. The basic principle of treatment is a slow rewarming of the patient and this is best done by nursing the patient in bed at a room temperature of about 25°C (70°F) so that the deep body temperature can be allowed to rise gradually. Other methods such as rapid rewarming by immersion in a warm bath, although effective in young people, are not to be recommended when dealing with old patients. The vaso-dilation caused by this quick surface heating may lead to a drop in the core temperature and to disastrous circulatory collapse. The disadvantages of the slow method of rewarming the patient are that the hypothermia is prolonged and irreversible changes in the tissues may take place. With mild hypothermia, this is, however, unlikely. Other cases should be admitted to hospital where, although conservative treatment is still indicated, precautions such as barrier nursing, isolation and broad-spectrum antibiotic therapy can be instituted. Severe hypothermia demands specialist treatment and often admission to an intensive care unit. The outlook for patients suffering from severe hypothermia is not very good. Where the initial temperature is below 30°C the mortality is high.

Prevention

Hypothermia is basically preventable. Old people should live in warm surroundings and this should include not only downstairs rooms but also bedrooms. The ideal range of temperature is between 65°F and 70°F or about 21°C. The cost of fuel is sometimes a problem. Old people on Supplementary Benefit can get a special heating allowance. Central heating, of course, is ideal, particularly when it is automatic. Electric heating is also satisfactory but expensive. The work associated with coal fires and the danger of paraffin heaters make these two fuels unsuitable for old people. Windows should be closed at night and special attention paid to insulation. Double glazing, draught exclusion and roof insulation not only help to reduce the size of the fuel bill but add greatly to comtort. If it is impossible to heat the whole house it is better in the winter for the old person to live in one room and bring the bed down to the sitting room which can then be kept at a reasonable temperature. People should be well clothed in bed; night caps and bed socks may not be such a bad idea. Electric blankets are useful, but may be dangerous if the patient is incontinent. Specially waterproofed electric blankets and low-voltage over-blankets, which use very little electricity and are safe, are now available.

Medical and social workers should be alert to the possibility of hypothermia and be aware of the people especially at risk. This could include all those over 75 and those living alone. There seems to be a certain section of the elderly community who have an idiopathic reduction in the body temperature stabilising mechanism. The problem is recognising these people. Perhaps wider use of the low-reading thermometer might help. Doctors should always be alert to the possibility of hypothermia and be careful in prescribing drugs, particularly tranquillisers, to those at risk.

Blindness

Over the past twenty years there has been a change in the age prevalence of blindness. These days, most severely defective vision occurs amongst elderly people. Visual failure can be an important cause of loss of independence and result in social isolation. With increasing blindness, mobility becomes more difficult and an old person is deprived of hobbies such as gardening, watching television and visiting the cinema. Vision can be quickly and simply assessed by asking the patient if he can read a newspaper, watch television or recognise the details of the photograph or picture.

Comparatively few people become blind suddenly and there is likely to be a gradual deterioration of vision over several years. This is always due to disease and old age alone is not a cause of blindness. The commonest diseases leading to failing vision are cataract, macular degeneration and diabetic retinopathy. Sudden loss of vision, when it occurs, is usually due to acute glaucoma, occlusion of the central retinal artery or vein, or a detached retina. Chronic open-angle glaucoma produces gradual loss of vision. Many of these conditions are treatable.

Cataracts, which may originate much earlier in life, develop slowly and are often symmetrical. Successful extraction and later optical correction using contact lenses are possible in old people, but the majority are more happily corrected with spectacles as contact lenses are only suitable for the dextrous and motivated; best of all from the optic point of view and increasingly used are acrylic lenticuli implanted in the eye when the cataract is removed.

Senile macular degeneration with pigmentation of the macula is difficult to treat, although, as the periphery is not affected, complete blindness does not occur. Many cases of macular degeneration are helped by low vision aids, for example telescopic glasses or simple hand magnifiers.

Diabetic retinopathy can be halted to a certain extent by careful control of the disease. Partial ablation of the diabetic retina, either by light coagulation or laser therapy, is useful in many cases as it delays retinopathy by cutting down the oxygen needs, hence allowing the ailing vasculature to maintain the important central area. Clofibrate may prevent deterioration but does not improve existing visual failure.

Acute glaucoma presents usually as an emergency. The angle is closed in these cases and the second eye is invariably at risk, hence the need for prophylactic peripheral iridectomy. Early symptoms include blurring of vision and the perception of 'halo' effects round lights. Glaucomatous haloes are specifically rainbow-lined – the so-called 'rainbow rings'. Monochromic haloes around lights are common and meaningless. Vision is subsequently lost and symptoms vary from an ache to one of the worst pains in the whole of medicine. The intra-ocular tension is increased and the pupil is usually fixed, oval and dilated, rather than distorted. The chronic, open-angle type which occurs in old people is much more insidious in onset. The visual field is lost, often to a remarkable extent, before the situation is recognised. It is important that this loss should be appreciated as it may be highly dangerous to old people, for instance, when crossing roads. Apart from field loss and raised intraocular pressure, cupping of the optic disc is present. When examining old people it is useful to check the ocular tension and do a simple visual field test. Sometimes the condition is genetically determined and relatives of patients with glaucoma should be examined. Treatment is specialised and surgery is recommended for acute glaucoma. In less acute cases Pilocarpine drops 2% and Diamox diuretic are often sufficient. Neutral adrenaline eye drops 1% (Eppy) are used for chronic open-angled glaucoma.

Despite treatment, many patients with these conditions become permanently partially sighted or blind. Even in these cases, much can be done to help. The first essential is to place the patient's name on the Blind Register. A certificate of registration (BD8 in England and Wales and BP1 in Scotland) must first be completed by a consultant ophthalmologist and forwarded to the local Social Services Department.

A social worker then interviews the blind person to explain the voluntary nature of registration and the benefits available. For registration it is necessary to define blindness and partial-sightedness. The criteria for these are summarised in Tables 17.2 and 17.3. These are fully set out on Form BD8.

The statutory definition for the purposes of registration as a blind person under the National Assistance Act of 1948 is that the person is so blind as to be unable to perform any work for which eyesight is essential. This involves special interpretation as far as the elderly are concerned.

The principal condition tested is visual acuity but contraction of the visual field is also important. Three groups are defined: visual acuity below 3/60 Snellen, between 3/60 and 6/60 Snellen and 6/60 Snellen and above.

Group 1 – Below 3/60 Snellen

In general, a person with visual acuity below 3/60 Snellen may be regarded as blind. In many cases, however, it is desirable to test the vision at one metre and not to regard a person having acuity of 1/18 Snellen as blind unless there is also considerable restriction of the visual field. (Note: 1/18 indicates a slightly better acuity than 3/60, but as the standard test types provide a line of letters which one possessed of full acuity should read at 18 metres, there is some convenience in specifying 1/18.)

Group 2 – 3/60, but below 6/60 Snellen

A person with visual acuity of 3/60 but less than 6/60 Snellen:

(a) may be regarded as blind if the field of vision is considerably contracted, but
(b) should not be regarded as blind if the visual defect is of long standing and is unaccompanied by any material contraction of the field of vision, e.g. in cases of congenital nystagmus, albinism, myopia, etc.

Group 3 – 6/60 Snellen or above

A person with a visual acuity of 6/60 Snellen or better should ordinarily not be regarded as blind. He may, however, be regarded as blind if the field of vision is markedly contracted in the greater part of its extent, and particularly if the contraction is in the lower part of the field; but a person suffering from homonymous or bi-temporal hemianopia

Table 17.2: Categories of Visual Loss Indicating Blindness

Visual Acuity on Snellen Scale (corrected)	Field
Below 3/60	No other condition
3/60–6/60	Contracted field
6/60 or above	Field markedly contracted, in particular the lower part

Source: Tony Aston, 'Rehabilitation Today: The Newly Blind', in Stephen Mattingly (ed.), *Rehabilitation Today* (London, Update Books, 1977), p.131.

Table 17.3: Criteria for Registration as Partially Sighted

Visual Acuity on Snellen Scale (corrected)	Field
3/60–6/60	Full field
Up to 6/24	Moderate contraction of field
6/18 or even better	Gross field defect

Source: Aston, 'Rehabilitation Today'.

retaining central visual acuity of 6/18 or better is not to be regarded as blind.

Form BD8 also enlarges on partial sightedness and gives the following notes:

1. There is no statutory definition in the National Assistance Act, 1948, of partial sight, but the DHSS has advised that a person who is not blind within the meaning of the Act of 1948 but who is, nevertheless, substantially and permanently handicapped by congenitally defective vision or in whose case illness or injury has caused defective vision of a substantial and permanently handicapping character, is within the scope of the welfare services which the Local Authority is empowered to provide for blind persons – but this does not apply to other benefits specially enjoyed by the blind, e.g. Supplementary Benefit or income tax concession where eligible.

2. The following criteria should be used as a general guide when

determining whether a person falls within the scope of the welfare provisions for the partially sighted, as well as in recommending, where the person is under sixteen years of age, the appropriate type of school for the particular child concerned:

(i) for registration purposes and the provision of welfare services those with visual acuity –
  (a) 3/60 to 6/60 with full field;
  (b) up to 6/24 with moderate contraction of the field, opacities in media, or aphakia;
  (c) 6/18 or even better if there is a gross field defect, e.g. hemianopia, or there is marked contraction of the field as in pigmentary degeneration, glaucoma, etc.

Registration in working adults has considerable effect on the help they get with jobs and training, but this is rarely applicable to the elderly. Social Service Departments are responsible for social care of the elderly on the Register. Casework is available, as is help with travel, supply of white canes and 'talking books'. Rehabilitation centres sometimes cater for newly blind old people. Some voluntary organisations are particularly interested in the blind and their assistance should be sought.

Despite this help, many old people with failing vision find it difficult to cope. There is a limit to what can be achieved by re-education and perhaps it is wiser to aim at only realistic objectives. First, the newly blind old person should be encouraged to walk around the house, making sure that no dangerous objects are in the way. The furniture should always remain in the same place so that he can learn the way around and gain confidence within his own home. Dressing and undressing can be made easier by using clothes which have few buttons and making use of zip fasteners. Shoes should be slip-on rather than laced. Shaving can be undertaken by an electric razor and eating and drinking can be helped by special utensils. New interests can be encouraged such as radio, records and tape recordings. Talking books are helpful and for the partially sighted, books with large print can be obtained from most libraries. Good lighting is essential.

It is perhaps too late for most old people to learn Braille but there are simpler types of tactile reading such as the Moon system which may be possible. There is much sympathy in society generally for the blind and an old person so affected should be encouraged to persist in social activities and remain a part of the community.

Useful Addresses

Royal National Institute for the Blind, 224 Great Portland Street, London W1N 6AA.
Scottish Branch RNIB, 9 Viewfield Place, Stirling.
Northern Ireland Branch RNIB, Bryson House, 28 Bedford Street, Belfast BR2 7FE.
Welsh Branch RNIB, 14 Neville Street, Canton, Cardiff CF1 8UX.
British Talking Book Service, Nuffield Library, Mount Pleasant, Wembley, Middlesex HAO 1RR.
National Library for the Blind, 35 Great Smith Street, Westminster, London SW1P 3BU.
Moon Society Publications, Helmsdale Road, Reigate, Surrey.

Deafness

The prevalence of deafness increases with age. In the author's 1970 survey of over-75-year-olds, 9 per cent were effectively totally deaf.[8] Many more could hear only the shouted voice and were prepared to tolerate the disability without seeking help. Unlike blindness, deafness attracts little sympathy. This adds to the sufferer's problems and because of embarrassment, they may become socially isolated and even develop paranoid symptoms.

Very simple tests will assess an old person's hearing ability. The response to a ticking watch, a whispered, normal and shouted voice gives an adequate estimate of hearing. Loss of high-tone consonants occurs first and therefore it is necessary to exaggerate these when talking to a deaf old person.

The basic types of hearing loss are conductive deafness, nerve deafness and a combination of the two, mixed deafness. Rinne's test distinguishes conductive and nerve deafness. This is carried out by holding a vibrating tuning fork first close to the ear canal, and then immediately pressing the base of the fork on the bone behind the ear. It is heard better via the bone in conductive losses; the opposite is the case in nerve deafness (and the normal ear).

Wax and catarrh may only muffle otherwise good hearing but can considerably aggravate poor hearing. Catarrh can be treated by antihistamine preparations but a watch should be made for raised blood pressure. Good benefit is obtained by syringing away wax, which if hard, should be softened by a few days' use of proprietary wax-softening drops, e.g. Cerumol. When syringing, it is necessary to be sure that the water is at approximately body temperature. If too hot or cold it can cause troublesome temporary unsteadiness.

Hearing is dependent on the vibrations of sound waves being collected by the ear-drum and transmitted by the three small bones (ossicles) of the middle ear to the cochlea, situated in the inner ear which contains the nerve endings of the hearing nerve. Conducted hearing loss is due to disorder of the drum or ossicles. Two common causes are a perforated drum or ossicular adhesions, both legacies of infection. Another common cause is otosclerosis, an inherited tendency to new bone formation which interferes with the stapes, the innermost ossicle. Nerve deafness in the elderly is usually due to presbyacusis – a word meaning gradual degeneration of the cochlea. Noise-induced hearing loss from previous noisy work commonly adds to presbyacusis. Less common causes are trauma, inherited disorders, Meniere's disease and Paget's disease of the skull.

Annoying head noises (tinnitus) may accompany many types of deafness. In the elderly, it cannot usually be effectively treated, although if the noise is pulsatile rather than steady, a check-up may be necessary. Explanation and reassurance concerning its benign nature help most patients to come to terms with the condition.

Hearing Aids

Behind-the-ear aids may help, but more severe deafness may need the greater power of body-worn aids (see Figure 17.1). Both are available to the elderly on the National Health Service. Very substantial help is given to most deaf people by these aids, but normal hearing cannot always be fully restored. Conductive deafness responds rather better than nerve deafness. It is essential to make sure that the old person knows how to use the device and a certain degree of teaching is necessary to bring maximum benefit. This is normally given at the hospital hearing-aid clinics, which supply a booklet called *General Guidance for Hearing Aid Users*, also available from the DHSS.[9] For those interested in further study, *Deafness*, by John Ballantyne, is an excellent and inexpensive guide.[10]

Figure 17.1: Types of Hearing Aid (Reproduced by Permission of the Controller of Her Majesty's Stationery Office)

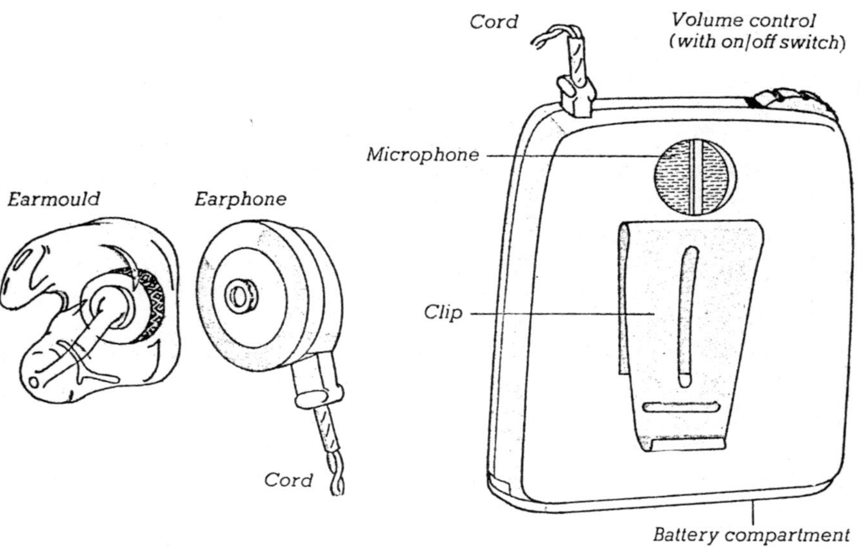

A typical body–worn hearing aid

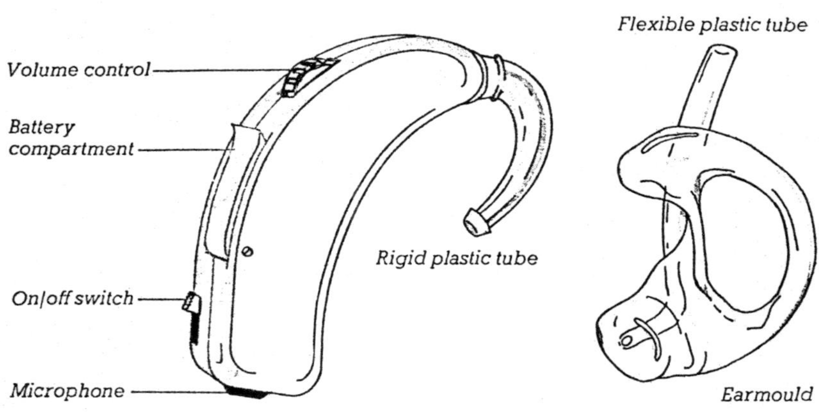

A typical behind–the–ear hearing aid

Notes

1. Bransby and Osborne, 'Social and Food Survey of Elderly Living Alone or as Married Couples'. *British Journal of Nutrition*, no.7 (1952), pp.160-80.

2. Exton-Smith and Stanton, *Report of Investigation into the Diets of Elderly Women Living Alone* (King Edward Hospital Fund for London, 1965).

3. 'Nutritional Survey for the Elderly', Report by the Panel on Nutrition of the Elderly, DHSS Reports on Health and Social Subjects, No.3 (London, HMSO, 1972).

4. *Recommended Intakes of Nutrients for the United Kingdom*, DHSS Reports on Public Health and Medical Subjects, No.120 (London, HMSO,1969).

5. H.E. Hyams, 'Nutrition of the Elderly', *Modern Geriatrics*, vol.3, no.7 (1973), pp.352-9.

6. H. Duguid, R.G. Simpson and J.M. Stowers, *Lancet*, no.2 (1961), p.1213.

7. Royal College of Physicians of London, *Report of Committee on Accidental Hypothermia* (1966).

8. E.I. Williams *et al.*, 'Sociomedical Survey of Patients over 75 in General Practice', *British Medical Journal*, vol.2 (1972), pp.445-8.

9. *General Guidance for Hearing Aid Users*, HAI Rev. Dept. of Health and Social Security.

10. John Ballantyne, *Deafness*, 3rd edition (London and Edinburgh, Churchill Livingstone, 1977).

18 THE CARE OF THE DYING

Death is the logical end to old age and the care of the dying old person marks the end of the services provided by the doctor through the ageing process. Many other people are necessarily involved, but at this stage the role of the doctor is usually crucial. Often, the relationships which have been built up between him and his patient over the years have turned to friendship and nursing an old person to his death after a long and interesting life should be a fulfilling experience. Sadly, it is becoming less common for old people to die in their homes (only 40 per cent do so), and these days most people die in hospital. However, deaths do still occur at home and the general practitioner and his team are called upon to manage these. In old age the commonest illnesses encountered in the community which lead to death are heart failure, stroke and cancer. All three can be associated with broncho-pneumonia, the traditional old man's friend.

The Function of the Doctor

The doctor has four main tasks when confronted with a dying patient. First, he must establish the diagnosis, secondly, he must alleviate distress, thirdly, he must support the family, and finally, he should co-ordinate other services. These apply of course to all ages and not just to the very old.

Diagnosis

It is necessary to be absolutely certain that the diagnosis is correct and that death is inevitable. A doctor must not only satisfy himself as to the incurable and fatal nature of the ilness, but he must also satisfy the relatives. If there is any doubt, second opinion should be taken; but if possible, subjection of a weary old person to intensive investigations should be avoided. Once everyone has faith in the correctness of the diagnosis and the eventual outcome, it is surprising how much easier management becomes. Nothing is more difficult than a family who will not accept the inevitable.

Emotional and Spiritual State

Most people fear death, or at least the act of dying, but many elderly people regard death with philosophical resignation rather than anger and frustration. 'I've had enough doctor, and I'm ready to go' has been said many times by the very old, and death is often a quick and happy event.

However, with a younger patient real emotional and spiritual problems and dilemmas sometimes confront the doctor. His previous knowledge of the personality may help him to understand some of these, and the doctor should always be prepared to discuss fears and anxieties. Family doctors are often in a special position to recognise these because of their previous experience of the person's emotional reaction to illness. Even though dying, he still remains a living individual human being and deserves to be treated as such. The real test of a relationship comes, however, when the decision has to be taken as to whether or not to tell the patient that his illness is in fact terminal. The decision rests on circumstances. Sometimes it is unnecessary to say anything and this is true in particular of the elderly, because they are often aware that life is slipping away. They know and accept that death is inevitable and this should be respected. There is a silent understanding between patient and doctor, and both realise what is happening. In other cases, particularly involving younger people, it may be apparent that the patient is reluctant to face the reality and does not want to know the truth. In these situations the doctor should tactfully avoid telling the full facts, but at the same time being careful not to destroy trust by making statements which lack credibility. Much can be done by discussing the causation of symptoms and making sure that they are effectively relieved. This course is possibly the most frequent one taken and it may be that it is unnecessary and cruel to spell out in precise terms to the patient that he is really dying. The wishes of the relatives should be known to the doctor and if silence is desired, all should observe this code. However, if someone really wants and needs to know the full nature of his illness and its likely course, particularly if his mental and emotional state is balanced, I personally think that the truth should be told. A person often needs this knowledge to make certain adjustments and prepare himself for the inevitable. Maybe certain relationships need to be re-established; he may need to come to terms with his past life and be happy with the arrangements made for family and friends. Judging when to tell may be difficult. Someone dying may go through distinct emotional changes. He may at first show a strong disbelief that anything of serious consequence is happening, and it is at this stage that pressures are brought to bear on the doctor for second opinion and hospital admission. This stage is often followed by anger and this is sometimes directed against the doctor who is held responsible in some way for the illness and its incurable nature. Linked with this are the emotions of depression and fear as the patient realises that his life is coming to an end. Gradually, however, there is acceptance of the situation and a more serene mood takes over. It is at this stage that the patient is perhaps ready for the whole truth and when he is prepared to come to terms with unresolved problems. This is an important stage to which old people particularly come to much earlier and they do not necessarily pass through the earlier stages described. Hopefully, eventual serenity is achieved and it can be an impressive and beautiful human experience.

Alleviation of Distress – Relief of Symptoms and Pain

The doctor has available a wide range of weapons for relieving distress and is aided in this by his nursing partners. It usually means palliative treatment of symptoms and adequate relief of pain. Mental problems also need attention. In younger patients, depression and frustration may predominate, but this is not as common with the very old and confusion may be the prevailing symptom.

Insomnia and Anxiety. Lack of sleep at night can be distressing to both patient and helpers. Sometimes there are physical causes such as bedsores or painful joints. These will have to receive appropriate treatment. The doses of all hypnotics in elderly patients need to be carefully considered and in the first place kept low. Tranquillisation and antidepressant treatment are occasionally necessary for anxiety and depression. Common preparations used:

Sedatives

Chloral hydrate Mist. BPC
Flurazepam 15 mg (Dalmaine)
Glutethimide 50 mg (Doriden)
Chlormethiazole edisylate 50 mg/ml syrup in 500 mg doses (Heminevrin)
Temazepam 10 mg (Normison)
Nitrazepam 2.5 mg – 5 mg (Mogadon)

Tranquillisers

Chlorpromazine hydrochloride 25 mg (Largactil) (can be used as tablets, syrup or suppository)
Promazine hydrochloride 25 mg (Sparine) (can be used as tablets or suspension)

Diazepam 2 mg, 5 mg or 10 mg (Valium)
Chlordiazepoxide 5 mg, 10 mg or 25 mg (Librium)
Thioridiazine hydrochloride 10 mg, 25 mg or 50 mg (Melleril)

Anti-depressants

Amitriptyline hydrochloride 10 mg t.d.s (Tryptizol)
Dothiepin 25 mg (Prothiaden)

Cough. A troublesome cough may be settled with a sedative cough linctus but it may indicate the presence of a chest infection. Occasionally a pleural effusion may be responsible for cough and will need aspiration. There is controversy about the desirability of treating terminal broncho-pneumonia. On its own or if it is producing distressing symptoms, it is necessary to give antibiotic therapy, but this may not be the case if it is the terminal event in another disease.

Common cough preparations

Linctus pholcodeine BPC
Linctus methadone hydrochloride (Physeptone) BPC
Elix. Promethazine BPC (Phenergan)

Nausea and Vomiting. There are many preparations for relieving these symptoms. Vomiting may be associated with other drugs or may be due to mechanical obstruction. Even when surgery is not contemplated, persistent intractable vomiting may require hospital admission for gastric suction and intravenous feeding. These measures are worth undertaking as palliative procedures.

Hiccoughs are sometimes troublesome and are helped by chlorpromazine hydrochloride in doses of 25 mg every 4 hours. Other preparations which are helpful in the relief of nausea and vomiting are:

Metoclopramide monhydrochloride 10 mg (Maxolon)
Promethazine theoclate 2.5 mg (Avomine)
Chlorpromazine hydrochloride 25 mg (Largactil)

Dyspnoea. Patients with heart failure or bronchitis are often disturbed by persistent and severe breathlessness. Apart from treating the disease itself, steroids (usually as prednisolone 5 mg every 4 hours) are useful for a short period and can be combined with diuretics and broncho-dilators. Aminophylline suppositories are often used to relieve breathlessness at night. Oxygen may be comforting and a cylinder can be supplied by chemists through the National Health Service.

Sore Mouth. Part of the general nursing care is attention to oral hygiene. Dry, sore mouths can be helped by regular washouts with glycothymol mouthwash or a proprietary preparation such as Oraldene.

Relief of Pain. Pain is perhaps not such a dominant symptom as might be imagined in a dying old person, even when widespread cancer is present. Where it is present, however, it demands efficient relief. Relieving severe intractable pain requires skill as well as drugs. Dr Cecily Saunders of St Christopher's Hospice, London, whose teaching has contributed greatly to the subject of pain control, believes that the key to success is constant control of the pain. This means giving the most effective drugs on a regular fixed routine. She aims to control the pain and then never allow it to break through again. The drugs should be preferably given by mouth, although injection may sometimes be necessary. A wide range of preparations is available and patients vary in their response to particular drugs and dosage. It is wise for a doctor to select a few analgesics and learn to understand their effect. Their action can sometimes usefully be augmented by other drugs such as tranquillisers. Where the pain is intractable and the patient is terminal oral heroin is sometimes recommended for relief as it has fewer side-effects than morphine and addiction in this type of patient is of no significance. The dose needed is 10 mg by mouth. Omnopon tablets 10 mg (Papaveritum) are also useful and may be more easily available than heroin. Various neurosurgical procedures are available for treating intractable pain, but these are seldom considered when treating a patient at home. Some neurosurgeons are prepared, however, to take the patients into hospital for a short period to carry out peripheral nerve blocks. Commonly used preparations for the relief of pain are:

Mild pain:	Paracetamol (Panadol)
	Aspirin and its allies
	Distalgesic (Dextropropoxyphene hydrochloride 32.5 mg, Paracetamol 325 mg)
Medium pain:	Pentazocine hydrochloride 25 mg (Fortral)
	Dihydrocodeine tartrate 30 mg (DF 118)
	Dextromoramide 5-10 mg (Palfium)
Severe pain:	Pethidine 50-200 mg
	Methadone 5-10 mg (Physeptone)
	Diamorphine 5-10 mg

Support for the Family

Apart from the patient, the doctor is faced with caring for the relatives. Even with a very elderly person it is sometimes hard to accept that death is inevitable. The doctor must again reassure them that the diagnosis is correct and that no cure is available. Even so, disbelief is sometimes slow to be resolved, but acceptance of the situation is eventually achieved and much love then goes into the continuing care and attention given to the patient. Relatives need not only emotional support, but also practical help with the management of domestic affairs. Although about to die, the patient is still alive and needs a full range of services. The doctor is probably the only person in a position to arrange and co-ordinate these.

Other Services

Nursing. The nursing care for the dying patient is provided by the community nursing service. The general principles of home nursing are described in Chapter 10 and apply with particular regard to such problems as pressure sores and incontinence. Supervision of treatment and pain relief by injection is necessary and is also very much the nurse's task. Special problems such as disposal of soiled dressings may occur and arranging for this may sometimes be difficult. They should be burned if possible, but otherwise they can be wrapped in a polythene bag and placed in a dustbin. Special arrangements can be made with Local Authority Cleansing Departments for this type of disposal. Offensive smells and odours are also sometimes a problem, but fortunately modern deodorants and air-fresheners can overcome this. Nilodor air freshener is an excellent deodoriser. Quite often a 24-hour nursing care service is necessary and Area Health Authorities may be able to provide this in some areas. Where patients are dying from malignant disease, the Marie Curie Memorial Foundation, Day and Night Nursing Service is available for this purpose.

The nurse is very much involved in general support and encouragement to the family. By the very nature of the problem, a strong bond of trust builds up between herself and the patient. The family also becomes very dependent on the nurse and she should accept this in the knowledge that it is self-limiting. Once the patient has died, the nurse should attend to the body and dispose of soiled linen. Any unused drugs should be destroyed and equipment removed.

Social Workers. In this country social workers have not been much involved in dealing with the problems of patients dying at home. Any social problem has usually been dealt with by the doctor or his nurse, or allowed to remain unresolved. These days, with economic, social and family problems increasing, and the added number of old people living alone without adequate support, the social worker is increasingly likely to be involved. Practical assistance such as home help, laundry service, special aids and adaptations are often necessary. The difficulties involved, however, in managing this type of situation where there is no family help does often make it impossible for such patients to die at home and hospital admission becomes necessary. So, in a sense, this reduces the opportunity for social worker involvement. It may be necessary to provide social support for a family which needs to deal with such problems as finance, the care of children and the disposal of effects. Counselling of a particularly upset member of the family may well be an important contribution made by the social worker, although the doctor must also be very much involved in helping with this type of situation.

Other Help. Much help can be had from voluntary organisations in sustaining a family nursing a dying relative. Social workers are usually able to locate these sources of help. Neighbours and friends are often invaluable in giving relatives a break and undertaking such tasks as shopping. Ministers and priests should also be brought in at an early stage and can bring practical and spiritual help to the family.

Bereavement

A bereaved old person is usually one who has lost a husband or wife, although occasionally they can have lost a son or daughter. These cases may well increase as a consequence of people living to a very old age. Old women particularly are likely to have to endure the loss of middle-aged sons.

Loss of a spouse in old age can be a very severe blow. It is a time of great vulnerability and not uncommonly the death of the remaining spouse is not long delayed. Most people never really get over this type of loss, but reactions may vary. Some superficially seem to cope and when socially well adapted may even marry again. Others, however, become withdrawn, depressed, apathetic and socially isolated. They do not care for themselves and lose weight rapidly through not eating. It is surprising, however, that often in old age people become insensitive to the deaths of others and are merely grateful that they themselves are alive. Perhaps when it is the spouse who dies it is the loss of support and help with caring which is most important. Here the health visitor particularly can help with sorting out the problems associated with finance, domestic arrangements and housing. It is also important to encourage the bereaved person to be outward-looking and retain (or remake) social contacts. Counselling along these lines is very important for the survivor.

Conclusion

Finally, everyone who has to care for dying patients must also come to terms with their own attitude to death. For most, it is an event clouded with mystery and easily relegated to the background of consciousness. For the religious, it marks a beginning, but for the unbeliever, a dark uncertainty. How should doctors, nurses and social workers react to a patient's spiritual need? If they are religious themselves and know the patient's attitudes, perhaps they can be involved in giving spiritual comfort. But for most this is a difficult task. It is probably best to leave these matters to the professional clergy. Patients do get comfort from religion at this stage and turn to it sometimes for the first time in their lives. An understanding and kind clergyman can bring great benefit in this type of situation. Sometimes, however, patients want to talk about these matters with a doctor or nurse. They then can at least show human friendship by allowing themselves to become less objective in responding to the patient's emotional experience.

Patients know who are the ones that care and perhaps this is not merely understood from the words which are being spoken, but also by expressions on faces. This type of communication is vital and once established, lightens the burdens for patients, relatives and professional carers.

Further Reading

Ronald W. Raven, *The Dying Patient* (London, Pitman Medical, 1975).
Cecily Saunders (ed.), *Management of Terminal Disease* (London, Edward Arnold, 1978).
Elizabeth Kubler-Ross, *On Death and Dying* (London, Tavistock, 1969).
Richard Lamerton, *Care of the Dying* (Hove, Priory Press, 1973).
Colin Murray Parkes, *Bereavement* (London, Tavistock, 1972).

PART SIX: THE FUTURE

The story has really now been told. Caring for old people has been presented in historical perspective. A picture has been painted of normal living in old age and an attempt has been made to give an impression of the social and medical problems old people might encounter. The difficulties experienced by the caring services have been described.

The idea has been presented that it is the quality of life which should be the concern of the caring team and that help should be available when this is threatened or disturbed. Prolongation of life is not in itself an objective, but rather the achievement of health and social contentment throughout life.

How will care develop in the future? Possibly along the lines indicated in the earlier chapters. In the final chapter, this question will be examined, but with a look also at the deeper implications of providing care for the elderly.

19 CONCLUSIONS

The aim of this book has been to describe the problems of caring for old people in the community and to outline the facilities which should be available to help in their solution. In discussing the characteristics of illness in the elderly, and the special social and medical difficulties experienced by them, together with the problems of the caring services, it has become obvious that a new look needs to be taken at the pattern of care which is given to old people. It has been argued that a clinic for the elderly will do this and solve many of the inherent problems. It is essential to have efficient day-to-day care of acute problems, both medical and social, but the clinic can take this a stage further. It is fundamentally preventive and can help with such problems as unreported need, but it can also contribute to supervision of treatment, rehabilitation, resettlement and the care of special 'at risk' groups. Health education can also be undertaken. Above all, the co-ordination of activities to help the elderly and the attainment of successful co-operation between health and social workers in both the hospital and the community can be achieved. This is the central theme of the book. The clinic will not solve all the problems – nothing ever will – but it will contribute significantly to improving the standard of care for old people. Hopefully, it will help in reducing disability and in keeping old people in the community for as long a period as possible in a healthy and active state. This is going to be vital when the numbers of old people grow even larger.

There is no reason why clinics of this nature should not become widespread, preferably based on general practice and an integral part of the function of the primary health care team (as for instance are antenatal clinics). It is essential that care given to old people should be the same as that available for the whole community, and not segregated off into a specialised domiciliary geriatric service. The schemes outlined in the book are practical and, hopefully, realistic. Idealism is bound to creep in, but even under today's conditions in the community, the principles underlying the clinic should be achievable. The clinic might also be a focus for the development of new ideas about care, for undoubtedly these are necessary. The aim must be to preserve the best of what is already being achieved in the community and to extend it to include new concepts.

It is necessary to undertake research to improve the understanding of the problems of old age. For instance, it would be helpful to have further evaluation of the housing needs of old people, particularly the place and scope of sheltered housing. Communications need to be improved and it would be a useful study to find out how this can be done. Transport and maintenance of mobility are also areas which need investigating. Screening the elderly as a method of solving the problems of unreported need and vicious circle effects needs evaluation. Studies should be undertaken into the effect which screening has on specific populations, using control groups and also long-term longitudinal surveys.

The economic and financial implications of providing services for the elderly in the community also need further study. Projects are already being undertaken which are designed to gain information on the comparative costs of different forms of care for old people with defined levels of dependency in different situations. Further work on the effectiveness of alternative types of care should follow.

The modern dilemma of the diminishing availability of the family as a provider of care is probably one of the most serious aspects of the whole subject. The reasons why this should be are likely to remain for a considerable time and, if anything, become greater. Yet the family is vital and every effort will probably have to be made politically to help the families to fulfil their responsibilities towards their elderly. Society must understand that it must help and be in partnership with those providing professional help.

Having outlined the practical situation and made proposals for improving services, perhaps it is also necessary to mention some of the deeper aspects of providing care for old people. It is most important, for instance, to know how they themselves feel about their own needs as there is a danger of younger people having preconceived ideas about these. There may be a discrepancy between how old people see their requirements and the ideas about these advocated by professional carers.

The quality of life anticipated in old age is subjective in nature and is particularly affected by the expectations and satisfactions of particular generations. These will change in the future and no doubt are changing now. There may well be mismatches between the services provided and those which people actually want. It is important, therefore, to know what society expects of old people and to relate services to how old people see their own needs. Many of the attitudes expressed by doctors and social workers are reflections of their own middle-class attitudes and may perhaps be unrealistic for a large section of the population. Certainly, old people today often want to be left alone and they value their privacy and independence. Obviously *adequate* resources for help are needed when acute situations develop and physical, mental and environmental comfort is important, but choice must remain if only to help old people maintain their self-esteem and sense of purpose. Many fear disengagement and yet society seems to encourage this. Continuing work and leisure activities are sometimes difficult to achieve and yet these are often vital in promoting healthy living in old age. How this is to be fitted into the modern dilemma of reduction of work due to labour-saving machinery needs clarifying. It would be helpful to have an idea as to how old people fill their time and to attempt to identify ways in which they could be usefully employed.

Above all, problems need to be seen in context. It must be continually asked, 'Who is this a problem for?' It may not exist at all except in the mind of the observer and is merely a phenomenon inherent to old age. However, on a national level, where real problems do exist, is it likely that they will be solved, and in particular will the challenge posed by the population explosion of elderly people be met? In some ways the situation is encouraging, but some doubts remain. On the bright side, it is true that services for the elderly are developing and expanding, especially in some areas, and there is evidence that changes in the pattern of care provided have reflected changes in real need. The expansion in the residential and domiciliary provisions which have occurred over the past few years has concentrated particularly on the over-75s and a greater proportion of elderly people now receive more than one service. The meals on wheels service is currently providing a more extensive provision to those who need it. General practitioners are becoming interested in screening their elderly patients and clinics are beginning to be established.

However, attitudes must change. Professional workers must fully realise the special problems which affect the elderly. Families and society must accept the responsibility for care. Old people themselves must integrate and not segregate. Retirement must not mean disengagement. The period between 65 and 75 must not be regarded as old age but rather as a golden opportunity for fulfilment and positive living.

Finally, the care of the elderly must not be regarded as the Cinderella of the Health and Social Services. Money and intelligence must be used to ensure the real needs of the elderly are understood and satisfied. In the community, the full resources of the medical and social team must be integrated and so organised that the lessons learned over the past few years are fully utilised to improve the standard of care given to our old people.

GLOSSARY

Aneurysm – A swelling of an artery caused by dilation of the walls

Anorexia – Loss of appetite

Aorta – A large artery arising from the left side of the heart. The aortic area is the part of the chest wall where sounds coming from the aortic valve can be best heard using a stethoscope.

Arcus senilis – A white ring round the edge of the cornea

Arrhythmia – Disordered rhythm of the heart

Arteriosclerosis – Thickening of the walls of arteries due to fatty deposits and calcification. Sometimes called atherosclerosis. A plaque means an area of arteriosclerotic thickening in an arterial wall.

Bacteraemia – Bacteria in the blood

Basal ganglion – Area of the brain deep in its structure

Bence Jones protein – Specific protein present in the urine in certain bone disorders. It coagulates at a lower temperature than albumen and redissolves on boiling.

Bradycardia – Slow heart rate

Chorea – A nervous disease, characterised by irregular and involuntary movement

Crepitus – A cracking or creaking sound

Decubitus ulcer – A bed sore

Dementia – Brain failure

Dermis – A layer of the skin

Diastolic blood pressure – Lower reading of the blood pressure when the sounds in the artery cease and which correspond to the resting phase of the heartbeat.

Dupuytren's contracture – A contracture of the fascia in the hand, causing deformity of one or more fingers

Dyspnoea – Breathlessness

Dysphagia – Difficulty with swallowing

Dysphasia – Difficulty with speaking

Dysrhythmia – Disordered rhythm

Ejection murmur – Abnormal heart sound with a characteristic quality

Embolus – A small body in the bloodstream which usually eventually causes a blockage in an artery

Embolism – Obstruction of a blood vessel by an embolus

Emphysema – Disease of the lungs characterised by distension of the alveoli

Erythrocyte sedimentation rate (ESR) – Measurement of blood viscosity which is increased in certain conditions

Epidermis – Outer layer of the skin

Faecal impaction – Blockage of faeces in the rectum

Fibrillation – Rapid movement of muscle fibres occurring in the heart to produce a rapid irregular pulse

Glomerlular filtration – Passage of blood through the kidney to produce urine

Grand mal fit – Epileptic fit

Haemoglobin – Red, oxygen-carrying pigment in red blood corpuscles

Hallux valgus – Deformity of the big toe

Heberden's nodes – Small swellings on the fingers seen in rheumatic conditions

Hemiplegia – Paralysis of one side of the body

Hypothalamus – Area of the brain

Infarction – Area of destroyed tissue resulting from blockage of blood vessel

Kyphosis – Curvature of the spine as in humpback

Multiple myeloma – Disease of the bone marrow

Myocardial infarction – Heart attack due to blockage of the coronary artery

Necrosis – Area of dead tissue

Neoplasm – A 'new growth', usually malignant

Occlusion – Blockage of a blood vessel

Oedema – Swelling due to fluid retention

Overflow incontinence – Inability to retain urine due to a full bladder and weak urethral sphincter

Paraplegia – Paralysis of lower half of the body
Parkinsonism – Symptoms of Parkinson's disease including tremor and rigidity
Presbyopia – Visual impairment due to reduced accommodation. Affects ability to do close work
Ptosis – Drooping of the upper eyelid
Pyrogens – Substances producing increase in temperature

Spurious diarrhoea – Diarrhoea due to constipation
Stoke Adams attacks – Due to heart block and characterised by a very slow pulse. May involve unconsciousness and convulsions
Systolic blood pressure – Upper reading of blood pressure, corresponding to contracture of the heart

Telangectiasis – Small area of dilated blood vessels on the skin
Tinnitus – Noises in the ear

Uraemia – Renal failure characterised by high blood urea levels
Urethral caruncle – Small fleshy swelling at the urethral orifice

INDEX